Strategic Patent and Commercialization Journey of Nemonoxacin:

From Molecule to Market

Chi-Hsin Richard King, Ph.D.

LCCN: 2026907823

ISBN: 978-1-971588-22-3 (Paperback)

ISBN: 978-1-971588-23-0 (Hardback)

Table of Contents

Prologue

The Story Behind the Story

Some moments in a scientific career feel complete - a discovery secured, a trial concluded, a drug approved. When I wrote The Journey of Nemonoxacin, I believed I had captured the full arc of a molecule that had shaped nearly two decades of my life. I told the story as I lived it: the chemistry that defined its identity, the pharmacology that revealed its promise, the clinical trials that tested its limits, the people who carried it forward, and the persistence required to shepherd a new chemical entity from concept to approval.

With time, I came to understand that this was only the inner half of the journey.

Behind every experiment, every regulatory submission, every clinical milestone, another narrative was unfolding - one shaped not in laboratories but in conference rooms, patent offices, licensing negotiations, and global regulatory systems. It was a narrative defined by timing, strategy, and the fragile architecture that determines whether a molecule becomes a medicine or remains an idea.

This second volume tells that outer story.

It begins where the first book ended: at the moment when Nemonoxacin stepped out of the laboratory and into the world. From there, it follows the molecule through the systems that would define its future - the patent frameworks of the United States, China, Taiwan, and Europe; the regulatory pathways that shaped its identity; the commercial landscapes that tested its value; and the life-cycle strategies that extended its relevance.

If the first volume traced discovery, this one examines definition.
If the first volume explored science, this one confronts survival.

If the first volume followed the molecule, this one follows the world the molecule had to navigate.

Together, the two books form a single narrative: the inner journey and the outer journey, the idea and its protection, the science and the strategy. They reflect not only the evolution of Nemonoxacin, but the evolution of my own understanding of what it means to guide an innovation from its first spark of promise to its place in the market.

This book is not a technical manual. It is a reflection on systems, on decisions, on people, and on the persistent work required to bring a scientific idea into the world. It is, in every sense, the story behind the story.

Chi-Hsin Richard King, Ph.D.
Saint Louis, Missouri
March 6, 2026

PART I

From Discovery to Definition

This is a story of inheritance, uncertainty, and the first strategic choices that shaped the molecule's future—a story that traces how a scientific legacy became a strategic puzzle and how defining "what we are protecting" set the tone for everything that followed.

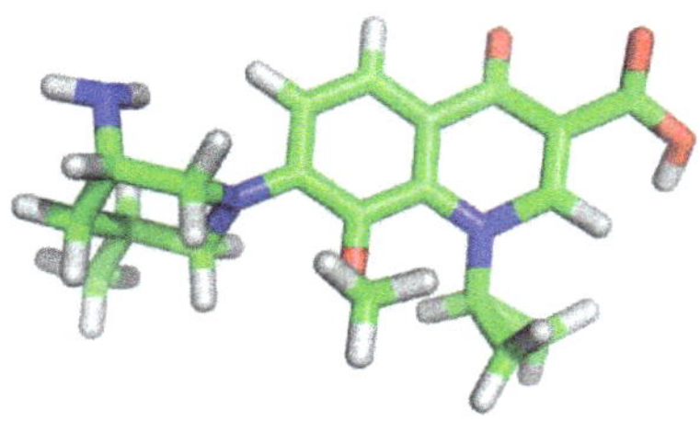

Chapter 1.

The Inheritance from Procter & Gamble

The Strategic Agreement That Started It All

The story of Nemonoxacin's second life began long before TaiGen ever saw a vial, a structure diagram, or a line of data. It began inside Procter & Gamble Pharmaceuticals, where a discovery team in Cincinnati had spent years exploring a bold idea: that a quinolone could remain potent without the fluorine atom at C-6—a structural element once considered indispensable. Their work produced a new series of non-fluorinated quinolones (NFQs), and among them, one compound stood out: PG-873870.

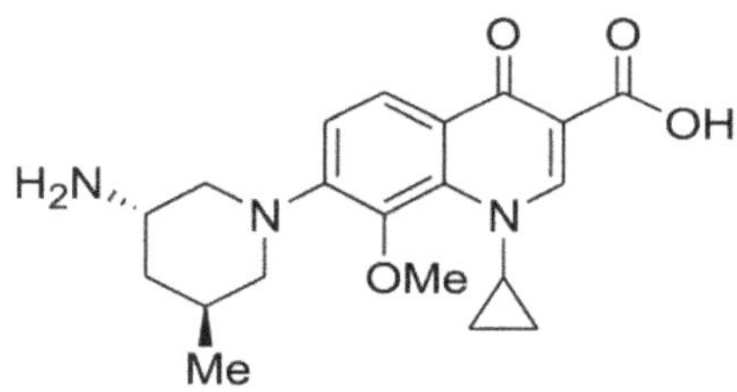

Chemical Structure of PG-873870

By the time the molecule reached TaiGen, P&G had already decided to exit the anti-infective space. The transition was formalized in January 2005, when TaiGen announced a strategic agreement with Procter & Gamble Pharmaceuticals. The deal was the product of months of evaluation, negotiation, and scientific review. On P&G's side, the alliance was led by Don Lucas, Worldwide Strategic Alliances, with Burrill & Company—represented by G. Steven Burrill—advising the transaction. On TaiGen's side, the effort was championed by Dr. Ming-Chu Hsu, President and CEO, supported by TaiGen's early clinical development, CMC, and regulatory teams.

The public announcement was concise: TaiGen would assume responsibility for Phase Ib and Phase II development, and in return would receive commercialization rights in China, Taiwan, Korea, and ASEAN countries, along with worldwide development rights through Phase II.

P&G retained the right to re-evaluate the asset after Phase II and determine whether to partner globally or resume development outside Asia. No financial terms were disclosed.

But behind the press release lay a far more complex inheritance.

Summary of the 2004-2005 Licensing Agreement

Parties:	TaiGen Biotechnology Co., Ltd. Procter & Gamble Pharmaceuticicals (P&GP) Advisor: Burrill & Company (G. Steven Burrill)
Date Announced:	January 6, 2005
TaiGen Received:	Responsibility for Phase Ib and Phase II developme Worldwide development rights through Phase II Commercialization rights in: • China • Taiwan • Korea • ASEAN countries

The Arrival of the Dossier

When the scientific package arrived at TaiGen, it came not as a polished development program but as a dense, technical archive - years of medicinal chemistry, microbiology, pharmacology, toxicology, and early formulation work. The dossier included:

- The chemical structure of PG-873870, a C-8-methoxy, non-fluorinated quinolone
- Multiple salt forms (malate hemihydrate, hydrochloride, anhydrous variants)

- Broad-spectrum antibacterial data across gram-positive, gram-negative, anaerobic, and atypical pathogens
- Mouse protection tests and pulmonary infection models
- PK studies in rats, dogs, and monkeys
- Resistance-selection experiments showing unusually slow resistance development
- CMC updates and early formulation notes
- US IND#68,976 for the PG-873870 Phase Ia study and the corresponding clinical report

The first time the TaiGen team opened the dossier, the impression was immediate: the science was strong. The compound's potency against resistant pathogens - PRSP, ERSP, MRSA, quinolone-resistant MRSA - was striking. The resistance-development profile was unlike that of other quinolones. The in vivo efficacy data were, in places, unexpectedly robust. The Phase Ia single-dose study in healthy volunteers suggests further investigation into safety, tolerability, and pharmacokinetics with multiple doses is warranted.

But the second impression was equally clear: the strategy was incomplete.

Interpreting the Inheritance

In those early weeks, TaiGen's task was not to innovate but to interpret. The team had to reconstruct P&G's intent from the fragments left behind:

- Why the 8-methoxy substitution was chosen
- Why the non-fluorinated scaffold was pursued
- Why certain pathogens were emphasized
- Why resistance-development studies were designed the way they were
- Why multiple salt forms existed without a clear development path

The scientific data gave confidence.
The gaps forced deeper analysis.

The inconsistencies made it clear that the program would need to be rebuilt - scientifically, clinically, and strategically.

The 2004–2005 agreement had given TaiGen the mandate to move the molecule forward. But it also placed the responsibility squarely on TaiGen to define what the molecule could become.

From Inherited Science to Strategic Responsibility

This chapter marks the moment when the story shifts - from what P&G discovered to what TaiGen had to decide. The inheritance was not simply a transfer of data; it was the beginning of a responsibility:

- To understand the molecule
- To protect it
- To rebuild its patent estate
- To define its development path
- To carry forward a scientific idea that had been left without a champion

In accepting that inheritance, TaiGen accepted the first challenge of the outer journey:

To transform a scientific legacy into a strategic foundation.

Chapter 2.

The First Strategic Question: What Are We Protecting?

From Data to Definition

The moment TaiGen accepted the dossier from Procter & Gamble, the scientific inheritance became something larger than a transfer of data. It became the first strategic decision that would shape every decision that followed - CMC, formulation, clinical design, regulatory positioning, and ultimately, commercial viability. Without a clear definition of the protectable asset, the molecule risked becoming scientifically impressive but strategically vulnerable.

The dossier was rich.

The patent estate behind it was sprawling, uneven, and expensive.

The Inherited IP Landscape

P&G's scientific archive was extensive, but its intellectual property footprint reflected the priorities of a discovery organization, not a development-stage company. The non-fluorinated quinolone (NFQ) series had been disclosed in publications as early as 1998. The core composition-of-matter patent family - P&G Case #6843 - had been filed in 1998 and had already spawned multiple continuations and CIPs. Several process patents existed, but many were tied to upstream intermediates rather than the final drug substance.

The Phase Ia study had been completed, but the clinical data had not been leveraged into any method-of-use or dosing-regimen filings. And several P&G patents - such as Case #6981, #8366, and #9007 - were already on a trajectory toward abandonment or low strategic value.

Patents Filed and Transferred from P&G

Entry	Title	P&G Case #
1	**Antimicrobial Quinolones, Their Compositions and Use** - PCT first filed in 1998 - US Patent No. 6329391 covering the lead as a new chemical entity - With CIP filings, a total of 5 patents granted in the US (US 6387928, 6849740, 7019143, and 7482254) - Granted in 37 countries	6843
2	**Process for Making Certain Benzoic Acid Compounds** - PCT, first filed in 1998 - Granted in the US (US 6348624)	6981
3	**Cyclization Process Step in Making of Quinolones and Naphthyridines** - PCT first filed in 2001 - Granted in 25 countries (CN1232508C, EP1343766, etc.)	8365
4	**Antimicrobial 2-Pyridones, Their Compositions and Uses** - PCT, first filed in 2001 - Granted in the US (US 6645981)	8366
5	**Antimicrobial Quinolones, Their Compositions and Uses** - PCT, first filed in 2003 - Granted in the US (US 6900224)	9007
6	**Process for Preparing Quinolone Antibiotic Intermediates** - The US first filed in 2003 - Granted in 11 countries (US6803469, etc.)	9009
7	**Malate Salts, and Polymorphs of (3S,5S)-7-[3-Amino-5-methyl-piperidinyl]-1-cyclopropyl-1,4-dihydro-8-methoxy-4-oxo-3-quinolinecarboxylic Acid** - US, China, and PCT first filed in 2007	10327

	- Published in PCT (WO2007/110834), US, and China in 2007 - US-2007232650-A1 - Entered PCT national phase	
8	**A Coupling Process for Preparing Quinolone Intermediates** - US, China, and PCT first filed in 2007 - Granted in the US (US 7456279) and Taiwan & Mexico - Entered PCT national phase	10328
9	**A Hydride Reduction Process for Preparing Quinolone Intermediates** - US, China, and PCT first filed in 2007 - Published in PCT (WO2007/110836), US, and China in 2007 - Entered PCT national phase	10329

The Strategic Context Behind the Portfolio

As we dug deeper into the dossier, another layer of complexity emerged - not from the science, but from the intellectual property that came with it. P&G had transferred a broad, discovery-oriented patent portfolio, much of which reflected the breadth of their research program rather than the needs of a company preparing to advance a single clinical candidate.

The portfolio included:

- Early-stage quinolone scaffolds
- Broad 2-pyridone series
- Upstream synthetic intermediates
- Multiple process filings
- Several antimicrobial quinolone families with overlapping scope

The First Act of Strategy: Trimming the Portfolio

This became one of our earliest strategic acts: pruning the inherited IP landscape.

We had to separate what was scientifically adjacent from what was commercially essential.

- The core PG-873870 substance and use patents were indispensable.
- The salt forms, polymorphs, and key process patents that directly supported clinical development were worth preserving.
- But the broader discovery-stage filings - interesting as they were - did not advance the path toward development, approval, or commercialization.

In 2006, TaiGen and P&G mutually agreed to reduce the portfolio to six essential patents, discontinuing maintenance on low-impact filings such as Case #6981, #8366, and #9007. This pruning was not merely administrative; it was foundational. It marked the moment when we stopped being custodians of P&G's research program and began shaping our own.

Looking back, the portfolio we inherited taught us an early lesson about identity and intention. P&G's filings captured the ambition of a discovery organization. But possibility comes with cost. Not everything we inherited was meant to be carried forward. Choosing what to keep and what to let go became an act of definition.

By narrowing the portfolio, we reclaimed control of our budget and sharpened our strategic focus. It was the first time we asserted what would become a defining principle of the Nemonoxacin journey: every resource must serve the molecule's future, not its past.

The Core Dilemma: Structure vs. Value

With the portfolio trimmed to its essentials, the first strategic question came into sharp focus:

Were we protecting a chemical structure - or a therapeutic value?

P&G's publications had already revealed the non-fluorinated quinolone concept. The 8-methoxy substitution was known. Even PG-873870's structure had been disclosed in scientific contexts. If

TaiGen attempted to rely solely on structural claims, the protection would be narrow, vulnerable, and expiring.

But the molecule's true value did not lie in its structure alone. It lay in:

- Its activity against resistant gram-positive pathogens
- It's unusually slow resistance development
- Its PK/PD profile supporting once-daily dosing
- Its safety potential as a non-fluorinated quinolone
- Its broad-spectrum coverage, including atypicals
- Its in vivo efficacy in pulmonary infection models

These were not merely data points - they were differentiators. And differentiators can be protected.

Reconstructing Intent from Fragments

To define what could be protected, TaiGen first had to understand what P&G had intended - but never completed.

The patent portfolio revealed a pattern:

- 6843 protected the chemical entity but was already aging.
- 8365 and 9009 protected upstream intermediates, not the final API.
- 8366 and 9007 were abandoned globally or offered little strategic value.
- No salt, polymorph, or formulation patents existed before 2007.
- No clinical-use patents existed at all.

The absence of downstream protection was not an oversight - it reflected P&G's exit from pharmaceuticals. Their filings froze at the discovery and early-process stage. TaiGen would need to build everything that came after.

The Strategic Reframing

The team began reframing the molecule not as a single chemical entity but as a platform of protectable attributes - a platform that could be expanded through new patents, new formulations, new clinical insights, and new manufacturing innovations.

The question was no longer:

What structure are we protecting?

It became:

Which attributes can be transformed into durable, defensible intellectual property?

The First Strategic Decision

The leadership team recognized that the molecule's future depended on a shift in mindset:

From inheriting P&G's science → to defining TaiGen's protectable asset.

This required:

- Identifying which P&G patents were worth maintaining
- Reducing low-value patents
- Creating new salt, polymorph, and formulation patents
- Filing new clinical-use and resistant-pathogen claims
- Building a manufacturing-based exclusivity strategy for China
- Ensuring that every development decision strengthened - not weakened - the IP estate

This was the moment TaiGen stopped being a passive recipient and became an active architect.

The Turning Point: A New Definition of Protection

By the end of the initial review period, TaiGen reached a pivotal conclusion:

We are not protecting a molecule.

We are protecting a differentiated therapeutic concept.

This concept included:

- A non-fluorinated quinolone with a unique safety rationale
- A compound with exceptional activity against resistant pathogens
- A molecule with slow resistance development
- A clinical profile supporting once-daily dosing
- A salt/polymorph strategy that could extend exclusivity
- A platform for new formulations, new uses, and new manufacturing routes
- A patent estate that could be rebuilt, expanded, and defended

This reframing changed everything.

From Question to Strategy

Chapter 2 marks the moment when TaiGen stopped being a recipient of P&G's legacy and became the architect of its future.

The first strategic question - What exactly are we protecting? - forced the team to define the molecule not by what it was, but by what it could become.

This was the beginning of the outer journey's strategic core:
to transform inherited science into a defensible, durable, and valuable asset.

Chapter 3.

Rebuilding the Patent Estate

From Inheritance to Architecture

Once TaiGen understood what it had inherited - and what it had chosen to let go - the next challenge became unavoidable: the patent estate around Nemonoxacin had to be rebuilt. The P&G portfolio had given us a starting point, but not a future. The core composition-of-matter patent (Case #6843) was aging. Several process patents were useful, but upstream. The salt forms were unclaimed. The clinical data had never been translated into method-of-use protection. And the global footprint was uneven, with many jurisdictions either inactive or abandoned.

If Nemonoxacin was going to survive as a commercial product, the IP had to evolve from a discovery-stage archive into a development-stage fortress.

This chapter marks the moment when TaiGen shifted from inheriting protection to creating it.

The Gaps Left Behind

The first step in rebuilding the estate was an honest assessment. The inherited portfolio had three structural weaknesses:

1. Aging Composition-of-Matter Protection

The 6843 family, filed in 1998, was the backbone of the entire program - but its clock was already ticking. Even with CIPs, the U.S. patents would expire in 2018. Europe, Australia, and many Asian jurisdictions shared similar timelines.

The molecule's scientific future extended far beyond the life of its original patent.

2. Lack of Downstream Protection

They are:

- Salt or polymorph patents
- Formulation patents
- Dosing-regimen claims
- Resistant-pathogen claims
- Clinical-use patents
- Manufacturing-route exclusivity

The absence of these filings was not a mistake - it reflected P&G's exit from pharmaceuticals. Their IP program froze at the discovery stage.

3. A Portfolio Built for Discovery, Not Development
Many inherited patents are protected:

- Early quinolone scaffolds
- 2-pyridone analogs
- Upstream intermediates
- Broad exploratory chemistry

These were scientifically interesting but commercially irrelevant. They did not protect PG-873870, nor did they support its path to market.

The estate needed to be rebuilt from the ground up - focused, intentional, and aligned with the molecule's future.

The 2006 Pruning: Clearing the Ground

Before new patents could be built, the old ones had to be trimmed. In 2006, TaiGen and P&G jointly reduced the portfolio to six essential patents, discontinuing maintenance on low-value filings such as:

- Case #6981 (benzoic acid intermediates)
- Case #8366 (2-pyridones)
- Case #9007 (broad antimicrobial quinolones)

This pruning was more than cost control. It was a declaration of identity.

We were no longer custodians of P&G's discovery program.

We were architects of Nemonoxacin's future.

With the unnecessary branches removed, the estate was ready to grow in the direction the molecule needed.

A Changing Ownership Landscape

Just as TaiGen began rebuilding the patent estate, the ownership landscape shifted again.

In October 2009, P&G Pharmaceuticals was acquired by Warner Chilcott, and with that acquisition came a new corporate steward for the original Nemonoxacin patents.

In August 2010, after TaiGen produced positive Phase II data under a U.S. IND, Warner Chilcott regained global rights outside TaiGen's Asian territories. For a brief period, the molecule's ownership was split again - TaiGen advancing development in Asia, Warner Chilcott holding ex-Asia rights.

Then, in December 2011, the landscape changed decisively:
Warner Chilcott transferred all worldwide rights to TaiGen.
With that transfer came:

- The complete regulatory package
- All related intellectual property
- Full global development, manufacturing, and commercialization rights

For the first time, TaiGen held exclusive worldwide control of Nemonoxacin.

What began as a partial inheritance had become a full one.
And with full ownership came full responsibility for the patent estate.

The Strategic Blueprint: What Needed to Be Built

Rebuilding the estate required a clear blueprint - one that addressed every vulnerability left by the original portfolio.

TaiGen identified five pillars of protection that had to be constructed:

1. New Composition-of-Matter Anchors

The original 6843 patent protected the free acid, but not:

- Salt forms
- Polymorphs
- Hydrates
- Solvates

These would become the foundation for extending exclusivity beyond 2018.

2. Manufacturing and Process Protection

To secure supply-chain control and block generic entry, TaiGen needed:

- New synthetic routes
- New intermediate processes
- New stereoselective steps
- New post-processing methods

These would later become the 2007–2009 process patents and the 2013 China co-development patents with ZMC.

3. Formulation Patents

The IV formulation, in particular, required:

- Stabilizer systems
- Solubilization strategies
- pH-control innovations

These became the 2008 parenteral formulation patent (60001-017001).

4. Clinical-Use and Resistant-Pathogen Claims

The molecule's true differentiation lay in:

- PRSP (Penicillin-Resistant *Streptococcus pneumoniae*)
- ERSP (Erythromycin-Resistant *Streptococcus pneumoniae*)
- MRSA (Methicillin-Resistant *Staphylococcus aureus*)
- Quinolone-resistant MRSA
- Atypicals
- Slow resistance development

These became the 2008–2009 method-of-use patents (60001-023001, 60001-024001).

5. Lifecycle and Regional Protection

TaiGen needed:

- China-specific patents
- Taiwan filings
- PCT coverage
- A strategy for global national-phase entry

This would later support the 2012 ZMC licensing and the 2013 co-owned China patents.

The blueprint was clear. The execution would take years.

2007–2009: The Rebuild Begins

The first wave of TaiGen-invented patents emerged between 2007 and 2009. These filings transformed Nemonoxacin from a molecule with an expiring composition patent into a drug with a multi-layered, multi-jurisdictional estate.

Salt and Polymorph Protection (2007)

Case #10327

- Malate salts
- Polymorphs
- Hydrates

This was the first new composition-of-matter anchor since 1998.

Process Patents (2007)

Cases #10328 and #10329

- Coupling process
- Hydride reduction process

These filings protected the manufacturing route and blocked generic workarounds.

Formulation and Clinical-Use Patents (2008–2009)

TaiGen filed five new patents:

- Parenteral formulation (60001-017001)
- Treatment of resistant bacteria (60001-023001)
- Pneumonia treatment (60001-024001)
- Antibiotic drug (60001-022001)
- Stereoselective synthesis (60001-025001)

These patents extended protection into 2028–2029 and established TaiGen - not P&G - as the primary inventor of Nemonoxacin's clinical and formulation identity.

2012–2013: The China Manufacturing Layer

When TaiGen licensed Nemonoxacin to Zhejiang Medicine Co., Ltd. (ZMC) in 2012, the patent strategy expanded again.
China-specific process patents were filed in 2013:

- Quinolone-chelated intermediate preparation
- Post-processing method for quinolone-chelated intermediate

These filings created a manufacturing-based exclusivity layer that would later become essential for protecting the Chinese market beyond the expiration of global patents.

2021–2022: The Final Layer - API Purity Patents Extending Protection to 2042

The last major evolution of the Nemonoxacin estate came nearly two decades after the original P&G filing. In 2021–2022, ZMC filed a new generation of API-purity patents in China and the United States:

China Patent (2021 Filing, Published 2022)
CN114437026A

- "Nemonoxacin malate API with low combination impurities and preparation method thereof."
- Filed: October 26, 2021
- Published: May 6, 2022

U.S. Patent Application (2022 Filing, Published 2023)
US20230201189A1

- "Nemonoxacin malate API with low combination impurities, and preparation method thereof."
- Filed: December 12, 2022
- Published: June 29, 2023

Most importantly, these filings reset the patent clock.
With a 20-year term from filing, the 2021–2022 API-purity patents extend Nemonoxacin's protection horizon to approximately: 2041–2042

This final layer completes the lifecycle arc:

- 1998: P&G discovery
- 2005: Transfer to TaiGen
- 2007–2009: New salts, processes, formulations, uses
- 2013: China manufacturing patents
- 2021–2022: API-purity patents securing the next 20 years

The estate is no longer a patchwork.

It is a fortress with a 40-year span.

From Patchwork to Fortress

By 2023, the Nemonoxacin patent estate had transformed:

- From a 1998 discovery patent
- Into a multi-layered global estate
- With new composition anchors, new processes, new formulations, new clinical uses, new manufacturing routes, and new API-purity patents extending protection to 2042

The estate was no longer inherited.

It was engineered.

The Strategic Meaning of the Rebuild

Rebuilding the patent estate was not just a legal exercise. It was an act of identity.

It marked the moment when TaiGen:

- Took ownership of the molecule's future
- Asserted its role as the true developer of Nemonoxacin
- Built protection that reflected clinical reality, not discovery ambition
- Created a patent estate aligned with commercialization, not exploration
- Ensured that Nemonoxacin would have a viable global life far beyond 2018
- Secured a final protection horizon reaching into the 2040s

This chapter represents the transition from inheritance to creation, from possibility to strategy, and from a molecule discovered by P&G to a drug defined, protected, and extended by TaiGen and ZMC.

PART II

The Patent Journey

This part becomes the intellectual and strategic heart of the book. It's where the reader sees how a molecule becomes an asset - and how an asset becomes a defensible franchise.

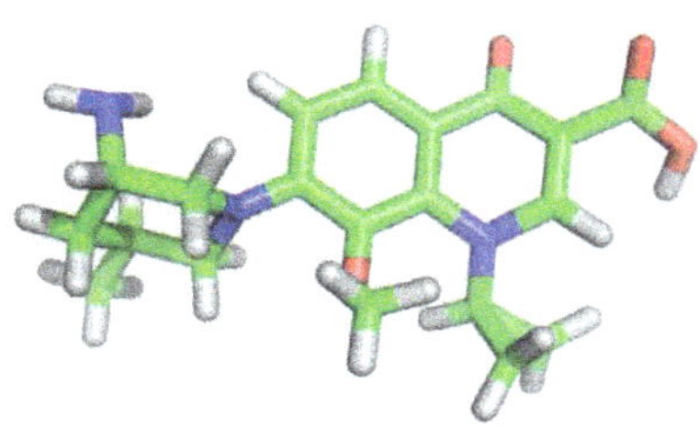

Chapter 4.

The First Layer: Composition of Matter

4.1 The Foundation of All Protection: Defining the Molecule Itself

Every pharmaceutical intellectual property strategy begins with a single, immovable anchor: the composition-of-matter patent. It is the legal declaration of existence - the moment a molecule steps from the realm of possibility into the domain of protected innovation. For Nemonoxacin, this foundational layer was not merely a formality; it was the structural core that enabled everything that followed: clinical development, global expansion, formulation innovation, and ultimately commercialization.

Before any formulation was optimized, before any clinical trial was conceived, and long before TaiGen existed as a company, the earliest architects at Procter & Gamble recognized that the molecule's unique structural and biological profile demanded broad, durable protection. Their foresight created the legal scaffolding that later allowed Nemonoxacin to survive competitive pressure, regulatory scrutiny, and international patent examination.

The story of Nemonoxacin's composition-of-matter protection is therefore not only a scientific narrative but a strategic one - a case study in how early decisions shape the destiny of a drug.

4.2 Structural Characteristics and Unique Advantages

Nemonoxacin distinguished itself from the very beginning. Unlike traditional fluoroquinolones, it is a non-fluorinated quinolone, a structural departure that proved to be both scientifically and clinically consequential.

Key Novel Features

- Broad-spectrum antibacterial activity

- Potent activity against drug-resistant pathogens, including MRSA and multidrug-resistant Streptococcus pneumoniae
- Absence of typical quinolone toxicities, including:
- Phototoxicity
- Liver toxicity
- Cardiotoxicity
- Tendinitis and tendon rupture

These advantages were not marketing claims; they were rooted in the molecule's chemistry. The unique substitution pattern on the quinolone scaffold - including the absence of fluorine and the presence of specific heterocyclic modifications - produced a pharmacological profile that was both powerful and safer than its predecessors.

Structure–Activity Insights

The early medicinal chemistry work demonstrated that Nemonoxacin could:

- Enhance activity against Gram-positive bacteria
- Retain activity against Gram-negative and atypical pathogens
- Maintain potency against resistant strains where fluoroquinolones were failing

This combination of breadth, potency, and safety formed the scientific justification for broad composition-of-matter claims - and later became the backbone of TaiGen's global IP strategy.

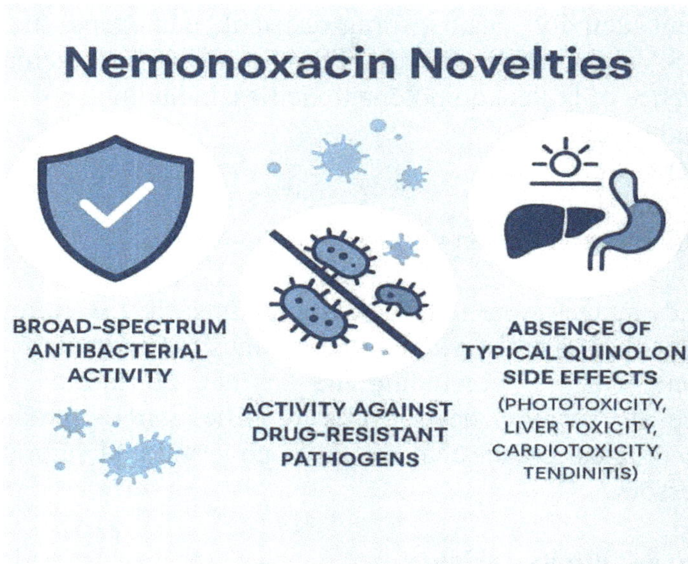

1. Broad spectrum of antibacterial activity
2. Active against drug resistant pathogens
3. No adverse drug reactions of other quinolones
   - Phototoxicity
   - Liver toxicity
   - Cardiotoxicity
   - Tendinitis and tendon rupture

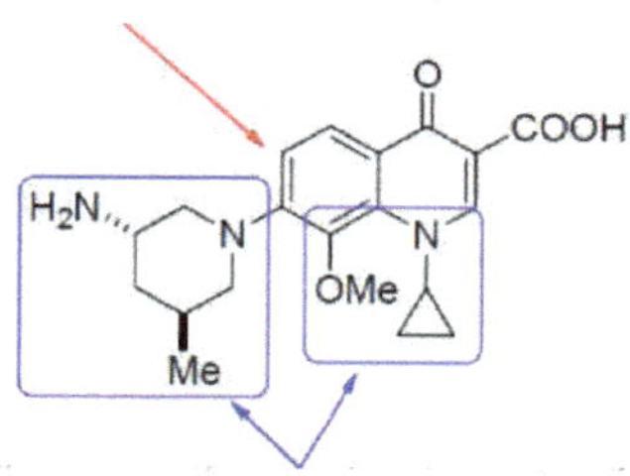

Enhance activity against Gram-positive bacteria.
Retain activity against Gram-negative & atypical bacteria.
Active against Methicillin-resistance *S. aureus* & multiple-drug resistant *S. pneumoniae*

4.3 The Provisional Patent: Establishing Priority (1997)

The first formal step in Nemonoxacin's IP journey was the filing of US Provisional Application 60/058,891 on September 15, 1997.

This provisional application:

- Disclosed a broad class of novel non-fluorinated quinolone compounds

- Included pharmaceutical compositions and therapeutic applications
- Established the priority date that anchored all future filings
- Provided a 12-month confidential window to refine data, optimize structures, and strengthen claims before public disclosure

This early move was strategically essential. It allowed P&G to:

- Secure the earliest possible legal foothold
- Continue internal development without revealing structures to competitors
- Build a robust data package to support later non-provisional filings

In retrospect, this provisional filing was the moment Nemonoxacin's IP architecture began.

4.4 The U.S. Patent: Composition of Matter Secured (1999–2001)

Building on the provisional, P&G filed the full U.S. application that became US Patent 6,329,391 B1, titled:

"Novel antimicrobial quinolone compounds, their pharmaceutical compositions, and therapeutic uses."

- Filed: March 10, 1999
- Granted: December 11, 2001
- Total claims: 53

Scope of Protection

The granted claims covered:

- Novel compounds defined by specific substitutions on the quinolone scaffold
- Optical isomers, diastereomers, and enantiomers
- Pharmaceutically acceptable salts, hydrates, esters, amides, and imides
- Pharmaceutical compositions containing these compounds

- Methods of treating microbial infections

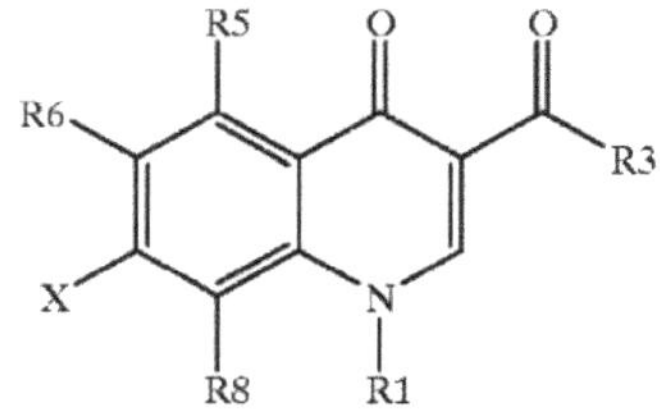

wherein:
(a) X is selected from

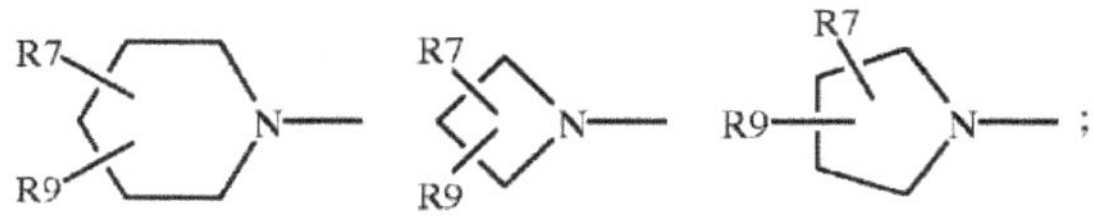

This was a textbook example of a strong composition-of-matter patent: broad, chemically anchored, and therapeutically justified. It became the cornerstone of Nemonoxacin's global IP estate.

4.5 International Expansion: The PCT and Global Filings (1998–2006)

To secure worldwide protection, P&G filed an international application under the Patent Cooperation Treaty (PCT):

- PCT/US1998/019138
- Filed: September 15, 1998
- Published as WO1999/014214 A1 on March 25, 1999

This PCT application enabled coordinated entry into major markets, including:

- China (CN)
- Europe (EP)
- Japan (JP)
- Canada (CA)
- Australia (AU)
- Korea (KR)
- India (IN)

- Mexico (MX)
- And many others

Ultimately, Nemonoxacin composition-of-matter patents were granted in 37 countries.

Taiwan Exception (1999-2004)

Because Taiwan is not a PCT contracting state, P&G filed a stand-alone national application, which was granted as:

- TW589306B
- Application No.: TW87115334A
- Filing Date: February 26, 1999
- Priority: US 60/058,891 (1997-09-15)
- Grant Date: June 1, 2004

Transfer of Rights

As part of the technology transfer from Procter & Gamble, the global rights to Nemonoxacin were assigned to TaiGen Biotechnology, forming the legal foundation for TaiGen's future development and commercialization.

4.6 The China Patent: A Case Study in Divergent Examination Standards (1998-2006)

Among all jurisdictions, China presented the most challenging path.

- China filing date: September 15, 1998
- Patent granted: July 19, 2006
- Patent number: CN 1264837C

The examination process involved:

- Multiple office actions
- Significant claim amendments
- Narrowing of certain structural definitions

Why China Was Different

China's patent examination philosophy differs from the USPTO in several key ways:

Topic	USPTO	CNIPA
Inventiveness Standard	"Obviousness"	"Inventive Step"
Claim Interpretation	Broader, context-driven	More structured, procedural differenced noted
Evidence Requirements	Flexible, evidence develops over time	Must present strong evidence early; no discovery

These differences ultimately compressed the original U.S. 53-claim structure into just four allowable claims in China:

Claim 1 - Core Markush Compound Claim
Claim 2 - Specific Compounds
Claim 3 - Pharmaceutical Composition
Claim 4 - Medical Use (Swiss-Type Claim)

The jurisdiction-specific constraints demanded careful strategic adaptation - shaping not only the final China claim set but also influencing TaiGen's broader global IP strategy in the years that followed.

4.7 Why the Composition-of-Matter Layer Matters

The strength of Nemonoxacin's composition-of-matter patents enabled:

- Long-term exclusivity
- Freedom to operate in major markets
- A platform for additional layers of protection (process, formulation, polymorph, and use patents)
- A defensible position against generics
- A foundation for licensing, partnerships, and commercialization

Without this first layer, none of the subsequent layers - no matter how sophisticated - would have been sufficient.

Composition of matter is the bedrock.

Everything else is architecture built upon it.

Chapter 5.

The Salt Forms: More Than Chemistry

How the malate salt became the second anchor of exclusivity

Salt selection is often described as a formulation exercise, a late-stage optimization step performed after the "real" invention - the active pharmaceutical ingredient - has already been secured. But for Nemonoxacin, the salt forms became something far more consequential. They were not merely chemical derivatives; they were strategic instruments, regulatory enablers, and, ultimately, the bridge that carried the molecule from discovery into a defensible commercial future.

By the time TaiGen inherited the quinolone scaffold disclosed in U.S. Patent 6,329,391 B1, the core composition-of-matter protection was already fixed. What remained was the responsibility - and the opportunity - to build the next layers of exclusivity. The malate salts and their polymorphs would become one of the most important of those layers.

Building on the core quinolone scaffold, TaiGen advanced into a new phase of intellectual property strategy: protecting the molecule not only as a chemical entity, but as a physical form. This effort culminated in a dedicated patent family covering the malate salts and polymorphs of Nemonoxacin's (3S,5S) isomer - an essential step in transforming a promising compound into a manufacturable, stable, and clinically viable drug product.

5.1 The U.S. Patent: Establishing the Salt-Form Family

The U.S. filings formed the backbone of the salt-form patent estate. The sequence began with a provisional application and matured into a full composition-of-matter–level protection for the malate salts and their polymorphs.

U.S. Patent 8,039,485 B2

"Malate salts, and polymorphs of (3S,5S)-7-[3-amino-5-methyl-piperidinyl]-1-cyclopropyl-1,4-dihydro-8-methoxy-4-oxo-3-quinolinecarboxylic acid."

- Provisional filed: March 28, 2006 (U.S. 60/786,483)
- Non-provisional filed: March 26, 2007 (U.S. 11/728,343)
- Published: October 4, 2007 (US 2007/0232650 A1)
- Granted: October 18, 2011
- Total claims: 17

The U.S. patent secured a comprehensive suite of embodiments:

- The malate salt of the (3S,5S) Nemonoxacin isomer
- Five distinct polymorphs:
- D, L-malate hemihydrate
- D-malate hydrate
- L-malate hydrate
- D-malate anhydrate
- L-malate anhydrate
- Characterization by:
- X-ray diffraction (XRD)
- Solid-state NMR
- Infrared (IR) spectroscopy
- Pharmaceutical compositions
- Methods of treating infectious diseases

This was textbook lifecycle management: a new patent family, independent of the original composition-of-matter patent, extending protection well beyond the expiration of US 6,329,391.
But while the U.S. system is generous to well-supported polymorph claims, China - as TaiGen would learn - was not.

5.2 The China Patent: A Parallel but More Difficult Journey

The flagship filing in China mirrored the U.S. invention but faced a very different examination philosophy.

China Patent CN 101045725 B
"某些喹诺酮化合物的苹果酸盐和多晶型物"

"Malate salts and polymorphs of (3S,5S)-7-[3-amino-5-methyl-piperidinyl]-1-cyclopropyl-1,4-dihydro-8-methoxy-4-oxo-3-quinolinecarboxylic acid."

- Filed: March 28, 2006
- Granted: December 5, 2012
- Total claims: 17

China required:

- Extensive experimental support
- Clear differentiation between polymorphs
- Precise structural characterization
- Demonstration of reproducibility and stability

Even with a robust data package, the Chinese examiners scrutinized every claim. The result was a granted patent with the same number of claims as the U.S. counterpart, but each one was tightly constrained and tied to a specific crystalline fingerprint.
Where the U.S. allowed broad conceptual claims, China demanded crystalline specificity.

This divergence reflected a deeper truth: China evaluates pharmaceutical salts through a lens shaped by its own industrial history and policy priorities. Novelty and inventiveness were judged more narrowly, and the burden of proof rested heavily on the applicant.

5.3 Why Salt Forms Matter

For a drug like Nemonoxacin, the free acid alone is rarely suitable for commercial development. Salt formation can dramatically alter:

- Solubility and dissolution rate
- Chemical and physical stability
- Bioavailability
- Manufacturing robustness
- Shelf-life and storage conditions

Selecting the right salt is therefore not merely a formulation choice - it is a strategic act of invention.

Among the various malate-based crystalline forms discovered, the D, L-malate hemihydrate emerged as the optimal API candidate. It offered a uniquely advantageous combination of:

- Exceptional solid-state stability
- Consistent crystallinity across manufacturing scales
- Ease of isolation from reaction mixtures
- Straightforward purification without complex solvent systems

These attributes made the D, L-malate hemihydrate not only scientifically attractive but also commercially decisive. It became the final selected API form for Nemonoxacin, anchoring both the regulatory filings and the industrial manufacturing process.

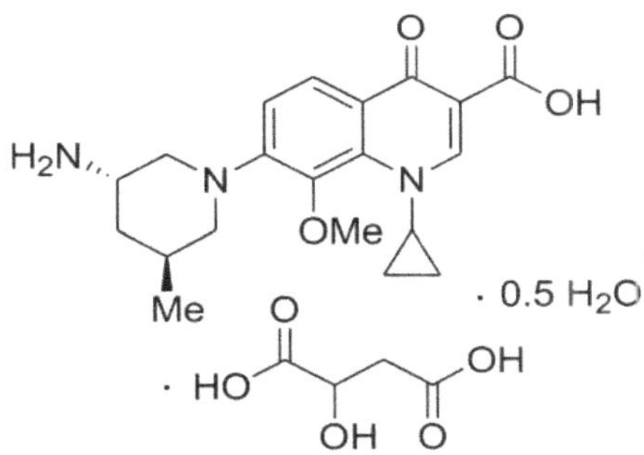

Nemonoxacin D, L-malate hemihydrate
Molecular Formula: $C_{24}H_{32}N_3O_{9.5}$
Molecular Weight: 514.53

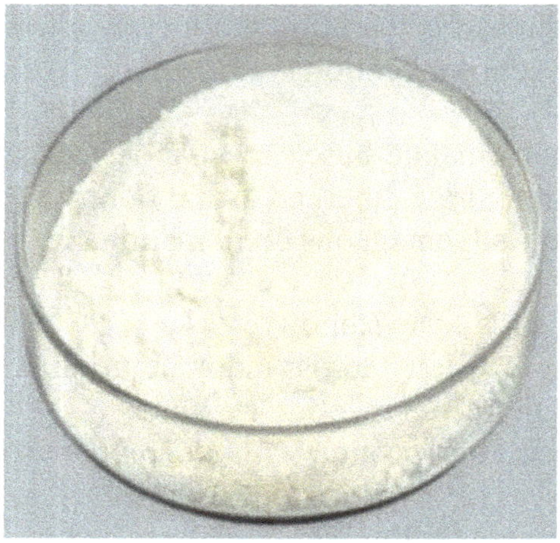

5.4 Scope of IP Claim Coverage

The malate-salt patent family (U.S. and China) protects a comprehensive suite of solid-state forms. The scope of coverage includes:

1. Composition-of-Matter Claims

- The malate salt of the (3S,5S) Nemonoxacin isomer
- D-malate, L-malate, and D, L-malate variants
- Hydrates and anhydrates
- Specific crystalline forms defined by analytical fingerprints

2. Polymorph Claims

Each polymorph is independently protected through:

- X-ray diffraction (XRD) patterns
- Solid-state 13C NMR spectra
- Infrared (IR) spectra
- Water content ranges

These analytical signatures serve as the legal boundaries of each crystalline invention.

3. Pharmaceutical Composition Claims

Protection extends to:

- Formulations containing any of the claimed salts or polymorphs
- Compositions with pharmaceutically acceptable carriers

4. Method-of-Use Claims

The patents cover:

- Use of the malate salts in treating or preventing infectious diseases
- Broad therapeutic categories including respiratory, urinary, skin, and systemic infections

5. Manufacturing and Crystallization Claims (Implicit in Polymorph Protection)

While not always explicit, the polymorph claims effectively protect:

- Crystallization processes that yield the patented forms
- Conditions required to reproduce specific polymorphs

Together, these claims form a multi-layered IP shield that is extremely difficult for generics to design around without altering drug performance.

5.5 The Science Behind the Strategy

The malate salt work required:

- Controlled crystallization
- Manipulation of solvent systems
- Temperature-dependent nucleation
- Seeding strategies
- Solid-state analytical chemistry
- Stability profiling
- Manufacturability assessments

Each polymorph had to be isolated, characterized, and justified as a distinct invention. The XRD peaks - 10.7°, 11.98°, 12.5° for the

D,L-hemi-hydrate; 9.3°, 12.1°, 22.6° for the D-hydrate; and so on - became the fingerprints of patentability.

But beyond the analytical signatures, the manufacturing behavior of each form became a decisive factor. The D, L-malate hemihydrate consistently crystallized with:

- High yield
- Low impurity carryover
- Robust filtration and drying characteristics
- Minimal polymorphic interconversion risk

These practical advantages meant that the D, L-malate hemihydrate could be produced reliably at scale, with predictable quality and without the need for exotic controls. This manufacturability profile ultimately positioned it as the commercial API form.

5.6 Salt Forms as a Second Layer of Exclusivity

By the time the malate-salt patents were secured, TaiGen had built a multi-layered IP estate:

1. Composition of matter (inherited)
2. Salt forms and polymorphs
3. Formulations
4. Methods of use
5. Process patents

The salt forms were the first major layer TaiGen built. They represented the company's transition from inheriting IP to creating it.

The selection of D, L-malate hemihydrate as the final API amplified this exclusivity. Because the chosen form was itself a patented crystalline species, the commercial product remained protected not only by regulatory data exclusivity but also by solid-state IP that generics could not easily bypass without altering drug performance or manufacturing feasibility.

In this sense, the salt forms were not just chemistry.

They were on time.

5.7 More Than Chemistry - A Strategic Foundation

Looking back, the malate salts were a turning point. They marked the moment when TaiGen stopped being merely a licensee of someone else's invention and began shaping its own destiny. The salt forms were the first major IP assets born from TaiGen's scientific and strategic efforts.

They were crystals, yes. But they were also:

- A statement of independence
- A demonstration of capability
- A foundation for regulatory filings
- A shield for commercial exclusivity
- A bridge to the future of Nemonoxacin

Salt forms are often invisible to patients and even to many scientists. But for those who build medicines - and the IP estates that protect them - they are among the most powerful tools we have.

They are more than chemistry.

They are strategy, time, and identity.

Chapter 6.

The Formulation Layer: Oral and IV as Parallel Paths

Two formulations, two regulatory pathways, one strategic purpose

Formulation work is often treated as a downstream technical exercise - an afterthought once the "real" invention, the molecule, has been secured. But for Nemonoxacin, formulation was never a secondary concern. It became a second axis of innovation, running parallel to the chemistry itself. The oral capsule and the intravenous formulation evolved as two distinct but strategically intertwined paths, each addressing a different clinical reality, each opening a different commercial door, and each demanding its own intellectual-property architecture.

If the composition-of-matter patent defined what Nemonoxacin was, the formulation layer defined how it would enter the world.

6.1 The Oral Capsule: The First Pathway to Patients

Patent Anchor: US 6,329,391 B1 - "Antimicrobial Quinolones, Their Compositions and Uses"

- Filed: Mar 10, 1999
- Published: Dec 11, 2001 (as granted patent)
- Granted: Dec 11, 2001
- Total Claims: 53

The earliest formulation work for Nemonoxacin was rooted in the medicinal chemistry program that produced the compound itself. The foundational U.S. patent - US 6,329,391 - did more than disclose the molecule. It also described the pharmaceutical compositions suitable for oral administration, including capsule and tablet forms. This was typical for quinolone development: oral delivery was the default route, the one that defined outpatient utility and market reach.

The oral formulation had several advantages:

- High bioavailability
- Stability in solid form
- Ease of manufacturing
- Regulatory familiarity

For TaiGen, the oral capsule was the first formulation to reach clinical trials and the first to define Nemonoxacin's identity as a next-generation respiratory anti-infective. But oral delivery alone could not address the realities of hospital-based infectious-disease management in Asia.

A second path was required.

6.2 The IV Formulation: A Parallel Innovation Track

The decision to pursue an intravenous formulation was not merely a clinical necessity - it was a strategic one. In China and many Asian markets, large-volume parenteral (LVP) solutions are a major revenue engine. Hospitals rely heavily on IV antibiotics, and procurement systems often favor products that integrate seamlessly into existing infusion workflows.

To participate in this market, Nemonoxacin needed more than a vial. It needed a stable, isotonic, ready-to-infuse solution - a formulation that could withstand sterilization, storage, and the rigors of hospital pharmacy operations.
This challenge became the foundation of a new patent family.

6.3 The Breakthrough Patent: The Malate-Salt Parenteral Formulation

China (CN) Patent Anchor
CN 101361739 B - "抗菌剂的肠胃外制剂 (Antimicrobial Parenteral Formulation)."

- Filed: Aug 9, 2007
- Published: Jan 28, 2009 (A-publication)
- Granted: Mar 14, 2012 (B-publication)

- Total Claims: 38

United States (US) Patent Anchor
US 8,658,183 B2 - "Antimicrobial Parenteral Formulation"

- Filed: Aug 9, 2007
- Published: Feb 12, 2009 (US 2009/0042932 A1)
- Granted: Feb 25, 2014
- Total Claims: 27

These patents captured the core innovation: the discovery that the D, L-malate salt of Nemonoxacin, combined with a carefully chosen isotonic agent, produced a stable aqueous formulation suitable for IV injection or infusion.

The invention protected:

- The malate salt form
- Isotonic agents (NaCl, dextrose, mannitol, sorbitol, etc.)
- Stabilizers, buffers, antioxidants
- Concentration ranges enabling LVP manufacturing
- Clinical uses across a broad spectrum of infections

This was not a narrow formulation claim - it was a platform.

The Global Architecture of the Formulation Estate

The international application WO2009/023473 served as the parent for all major national-phase filings in this formulation family, including EP2185143, JP5805389, TW I391135, KR101313858, CA2693041, AU2008287144, and ultimately US 8,658,183 B2. This single WO disclosure became the nucleus from which TaiGen built a coordinated, multinational protection strategy for the IV formulation.

6.4 Why the IV Formulation Became a Strategic Asset in Asia

In China, IV antibiotics dominate hospital procurement. Large-volume parenteral solutions - 250 mL, 500 mL, even 1000 mL - are routine. They are:

- Reimbursed differently
- Purchased in higher volumes
- Preferred for moderate to severe infections
- Central to hospital revenue models

For a new antibiotic, having an IV formulation is not optional - it is the gateway to hospital adoption.

TaiGen recognized this early. The IV formulation patent—especially CN101361739B - became a cornerstone of hospital-based exclusivity and a major commercial lever.

6.5 Parallel Paths, Unified Strategy

The oral and IV formulations were not sequential developments. They were parallel paths, each reinforcing the other:

Oral Capsule	**IV Formulation**
Outpatient Use	Inpatient Use
Early clinical trials	Severe infection management
Lower cost	Higher hospital revenue
Covered by US 6,329,391	Patented by CN101361739B & US8,658,183B2

Together, they created a continuum of care:

1. IV loading for severe cases
2. Oral step-down therapy for discharge
3. Unified brand identity across settings

This dual-formulation strategy is now standard for modern antibiotics, but for Nemonoxacin, it was a deliberate design choice made early, before the molecule had even completed its clinical journey.

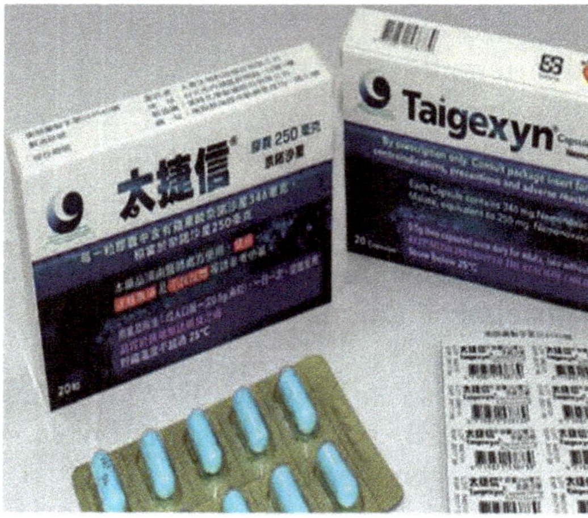

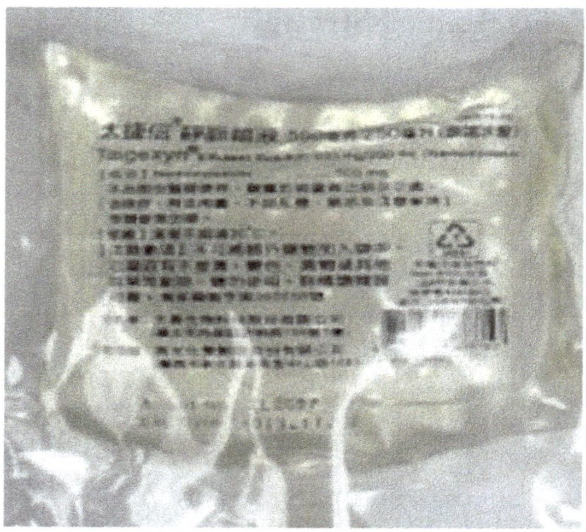

6.6 The Formulation Layer as a Pillar of Lifecycle Management

From an IP perspective, the formulation layer served several critical functions:

- Extended protection beyond the composition-of-matter patent
- Enabled new regulatory filings
- Created barriers to generic entry
- Supported differentiated labeling
- Opened new markets and revenue channels

In China, the IV formulation patent (CN101361739B) protected the hospital market through 2027.

In the U.S., the corresponding patent (US 8,658,183 B2) extends protection to 2031, long after the core molecule patent expired.

This is the essence of formulation-layer strategy:

A scientific solution that becomes a commercial moat.

6.7 A Layer That Reflects the Philosophy of the Whole Program

The formulation layer embodies the broader philosophy behind Nemonoxacin's development:

- Solve real clinical problems
- Design for the realities of global markets
- Use IP not as a shield, but as a structure
- Build parallel paths, not sequential dependencies

The oral and IV formulations are not two versions of the same drug. There are two expressions of the same idea: that innovation must meet patients where they are - whether in a rural clinic, a major hospital, or a home recovering from pneumonia.

In this sense, the formulation layer is not merely technical. It is architectural. It is the bridge between chemistry and care, between invention and impact.

Chapter 7.

The Method-of-Use Layer- Protecting Clinical Reality

By the late 2000s, the scientific story of Nemonoxacin had already taken shape: a non-fluorinated quinolone with a distinctive (3S,5S) stereochemistry, broad Gram-positive potency, and a safety profile that set it apart from its fluoroquinolone predecessors. But a molecule, no matter how elegant, does not become a medicine simply by existing. It must survive the world it enters - a world of resistant pathogens, shifting clinical standards, and competitors eager to exploit any unguarded space.

This was the moment when the clinical reality of Nemonoxacin had to be translated into legal reality.

The scientific team had demonstrated that Nemonoxacin retained activity where other antibiotics failed: methicillin-resistant Staphylococcus aureus (MRSA), penicillin-resistant Streptococcus pneumoniae, vancomycin-intermediate strains, clarithromycin-resistant H. pylori, and more. These were not abstract microbiological categories; they were the organisms that defined the global crisis of antimicrobial resistance.

To protect Nemonoxacin's future, we needed a patent layer that captured this reality - not in the language of chemistry, but in the language of medicine.

Thus emerged the Method-of-Use Layer, a triad of filings that together secured Nemonoxacin's therapeutic identity:

1. "化合物在制备治疗抗生素耐药性细菌感染的药物中的用途" (Treatment of Antibiotic-Resistant Bacterial Infections)

CN101618038B (filed September 26, 2008; granted December 7, 2011)
US 8,211,909 B2 (filed September 8, 2008; granted July 3, 2012)

These two patents - Chinese and U.S. counterparts - are true global equivalents. They share the same priority (U.S. provisional 61/077,293, filed July 1, 2008), the same compound, and the same therapeutic vision: Nemonoxacin as a new weapon against resistant pathogens.

They protect the use of the compound to treat infections caused by:

- methicillin-nonsusceptible bacteria (including MRSA and MRSE)
- vancomycin-nonsusceptible bacteria (VISA, hVISA, VRSA)
- penicillin-nonsusceptible S. pneumoniae
- clarithromycin-resistant H. pylori
- metronidazole-resistant H. pylori

This was not merely a list of organisms. It was a map of the clinical crisis of the time - a crisis that Nemonoxacin was uniquely positioned to address.

By securing these claims early, we ensured that Nemonoxacin's therapeutic value could not be appropriated by competitors who might attempt to repurpose the molecule for resistant pathogens. The patents framed Nemonoxacin not just as an antibiotic, but as a solution to antimicrobial resistance.

This was the first pillar of the Method-of-Use Layer: broad, pathogen-defined protection.

2. "治疗肺炎的药物" (Pneumonia Treatment, Treatment of pneumonia with defined human dosing)

CN101618039B (filed June 30, 2009; granted April 11, 2012)
If the first pillar captured the microbiological reality, the second captured the clinical reality.

Pneumonia - especially community-acquired pneumonia (CAP) - was the indication where Nemonoxacin's clinical development would begin. The patent, therefore, did something the earlier filings did not: it defined human dosing ranges.

It claimed oral administration of Nemonoxacin at:

- 2–30 mg/kg/day, with preferred ranges
- 3–16 mg/kg/day
- 7–12 mg/kg/day

Dosing patents are notoriously difficult to secure, but they are also among the most powerful. By anchoring Nemonoxacin to a real-world therapeutic regimen, the patent created a bridge between laboratory potency and bedside practice.

It also narrowed the indication to pneumonia caused by:

- methicillin-nonsusceptible S. aureus
- penicillin-nonsusceptible S. pneumoniae

This was the second pillar: disease-defined, dose-defined protection, aligned with the drug's clinical development path.

3. "抗生素药物" (Antibiotic Drug, The (3S,5R) isomer as a defensive API patent)

CN101628911B (filed July 14, 2009; granted May 29, 2013)
Nemonoxacin itself is the (3S,5S) stereoisomer. That is the active pharmaceutical ingredient (API) used in the clinic and in the commercial product.

But stereochemistry is a competitive battlefield.

A rival company could, in theory, develop the (3S,5R) isomer - not because it was better, but because it was close enough to ride on Nemonoxacin's clinical success while avoiding the composition-of-matter patent.

To prevent this, we filed a patent specifically on the (3S,5R)-Nemonoxacin malate, including its hemihydrate.
This was not a patent for our own use. It was a strategic block - a way to close off the stereochemical space around Nemonoxacin so that no competitor could enter the market with a "mirror-image" variant.

In doing so, we protected not only the molecule but the integrity of the therapeutic franchise.

This was the third pillar: stereochemical perimeter defense. Together, these three patents formed a protective arc around Nemonoxacin's clinical use - one that extended from resistant pathogens, to a specific disease indication, to the stereochemical space surrounding the commercial API.

This chapter tells how that arc was built.

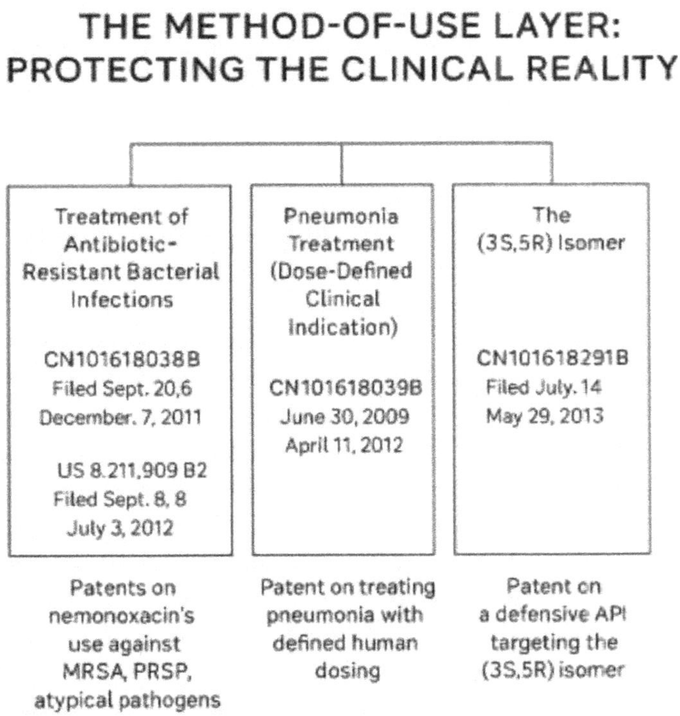

Closing Reflection - Protecting the Reality We Fought to Create

The Method-of-Use Layer was never just about patents. It was about **protecting the clinical truth** of Nemonoxacin - the truth that emerged from years of microbiology, medicinal chemistry, and clinical trials.

Each patent in this layer served a different purpose:

- One safeguarded the drug's role against resistant pathogens,
- One secured its first major clinical indication,
- One defended the stereochemical space around the molecule.

Together, they ensured that Nemonoxacin's therapeutic identity could not be diluted, diverted, or appropriated.

In the broader architecture of the Nemonoxacin estate, this layer is where science meets medicine, and where medicine meets law. It is the layer that protects not just what the molecule *is*, but what it *does* - and what it means for patients.

And for me, it is the layer that captures the heart of the project: the belief that innovation must be defended not only in the laboratory, but in the world it enters. The Method-of-Use Layer is where that defense becomes visible - a testament to the clinical reality we fought to bring into being, and to the legacy we sought to preserve.

Chapter 8.

The Manufacturing Layer: Protecting the Drug Supplies

The Quiet Power of Manufacturing IP - From early intermediates to the 2022 API-purity patents

Every successful antibiotic has two lifelines:

1. The molecule itself, and
2. The ability to make it - reliably, reproducibly, and at scale.

For Nemonoxacin, the manufacturing layer became more than a technical necessity. It became a strategic shield. By the mid-2000s, the composition-of-matter patent was already aging, and the clinical program was advancing toward Phase II. The question was no longer whether the molecule worked - it was how to protect the supply chain long enough for the drug to reach patients and sustain a viable market.

Manufacturing patents answered that question. They created a second perimeter around the molecule: a perimeter built not from new chemical entities, but from process control, stereochemistry, intermediate stability, coupling efficiency, and API quality. These patents did not merely describe how to make Nemonoxacin - they defined how to make it better than anyone else could.

This chapter traces that evolution: from early quinolone-coupling chemistry developed by Procter & Gamble, to TaiGen's stereoselective construction of the 3S,5S piperidine side chain, and finally to the 2022 API-purity patents that closed the loop by protecting the final quality attributes of the drug substance.

I. The Early Core-Intermediate Patents: Preparing the Battlefield

Before P&G's boron-chelate breakthrough, the foundation had already been laid by patents covering the preparation of key quinolone intermediates - the very building blocks that Nemonoxacin's manufacturing route depends on.

US 6,803,469 B2
Title: Quinolone Intermediates and Methods for Preparing the Same

Filed: December 20, 2002
Granted: October 12, 2004
This U.S. patent strengthened global protection for functionalized quinolone intermediates. It defined:

- The functionalized quinolone core
- Halogenation and activation chemistry
- Purification and crystallization conditions

CN 100406443 C
Title: 一种制备喹诺酮类抗菌药物中间体的方法
(Method for Preparing Quinolone Antibiotic Intermediates)

Filed: April 28, 2004
Granted: October 8, 2008

This Chinese patent covers improved methods for preparing 7-fluoroquinolone intermediates, including optimized halogenation, protection, and activation steps.

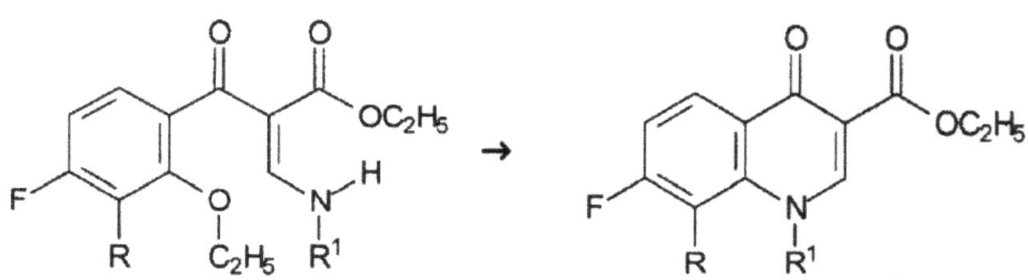

Together, US6,803,469B2 and CN100406443C formed the first moat: control of the quinolone nucleus itself. Any manufacturer attempting to prepare Nemonoxacin - or any related 7-amino-piperidinyl quinolone - would need these intermediates.

II. The P&G Hydride-Reduction Patents: Securing the Chiral Diol Precursor

The next layer of protection did not involve the quinolone core at all. Instead, it targeted the earliest committed step toward the 3-amino-5-methyl piperidine side chain - the stereochemical engine of Nemonoxacin.

US 7,528,264 B2
Title: Hydride reduction process for preparing quinolone intermediates

Filed: Mar 26, 2007
Granted: May 5, 2009

This patent protects a highly specific, industrially scalable hydride-reduction process that converts cyclic pyroglutamate intermediates into acyclic diols. These diols are the direct precursors to the 3S,5S piperidine side chain.

Key protected elements include:

- 2–4 equivalents $NaBH_4$
- 1.5–3 equivalents $CaCl_2$ or $CaBr_2$
- C_1–C_4 alkanol / C_2–C_6 ether solvent mixtures
- critical ratios such as 33:67 ethanol: MTBE
- temperature windows:
- –20 °C to 10 °C for $NaBH_4$ addition
- 5 °C to 15 °C for $CaCl_2$ addition
- safety controls preventing "sleeping reactions" and violent exotherms
- stereochemical and impurity-profile preservation

This patent is not about the quinolone core - it is about making the chiral diol precursor manufacturable at scale, safely, and reproducibly.

CN 101045695 B
Title: 用于制备喹诺酮中间体的氢化还原方法

(Hydride Reduction Process for Preparing Quinolone Intermediates)

Filed: Mar 28, 2006
Granted: Dec 15, 2010

The Chinese counterpart mirrors the U.S. patent and protects:

- the same hydride-reduction chemistry
- the same solvent ratios and temperature controls
- the same $NaBH_4/CaCl_2$ activation sequence
- the same diol intermediates

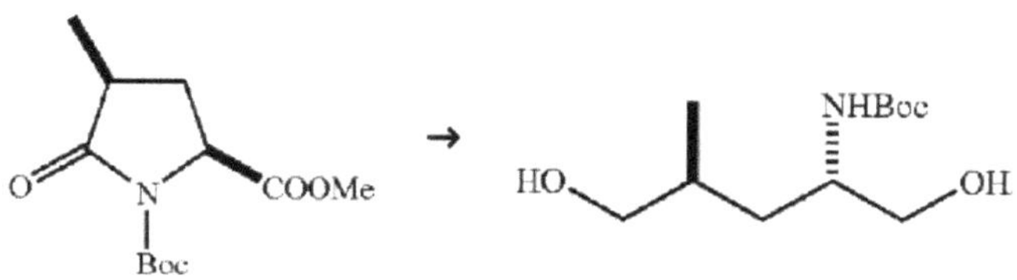

Together, US 7,528,264 B2 and CN 101045695 B form the second moat:

control of the chiral diol precursor that ultimately becomes the 3S,5S piperidine side chain.

This step is indispensable. Any viable Nemonoxacin route must pass through this diol.

III. The P&G Coupling Patents: Securing the Heart of the Molecule

Once the core intermediates were protected, P&G advanced the next step: coupling the activated quinolone with the piperidine side chain.

US 7,456,279 B2
Title: Coupling Process for Preparing Quinolone Intermediates

Filed: March 26, 2007
Granted: November 25, 2008

CN 101045724 B
Title: 用于制备喹诺酮中间体的偶联方法
(Coupling Process for Preparing Quinolone Intermediates)

Filed: March 28, 2006
Granted: August 17, 2011

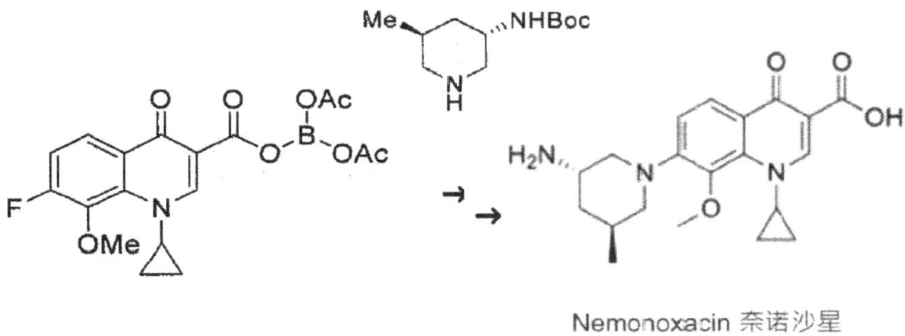

These patents introduced the boron-chelate activation strategy, enabling:

- Regioselective substitution at the 7-position
- Protection of sensitive 8-methoxy and 1-cyclopropyl groups
- Mild, scalable reaction conditions (20–80 °C)
- Clean coupling with Boc-protected piperidine

This became the third moat: control of the key C–N bond-forming step.

IV. TaiGen's Stereoselective Side-Chain Patents: Owning the 3S,5S Piperidine

With the core and coupling protected, TaiGen secured the side chain - the stereochemical engine of Nemonoxacin.

CN 102093260 B
Title: 哌啶衍生物的立体有择合成
(Stereoselective Synthesis of Piperidine Derivatives)

Filed: December 14, 2009
Granted: March 5, 2014

TWI386395 B
Title: 哌啶衍生物的立體有擇合成
(Stereoselective Synthesis of Piperidine Derivatives)

Filed: December 14, 2009
Granted: February 21, 2013

WO 2010/077798 A2
Title: Stereoselective Synthesis of Piperidine Derivatives
Filed: December 14, 2009
Published: July 8, 2010

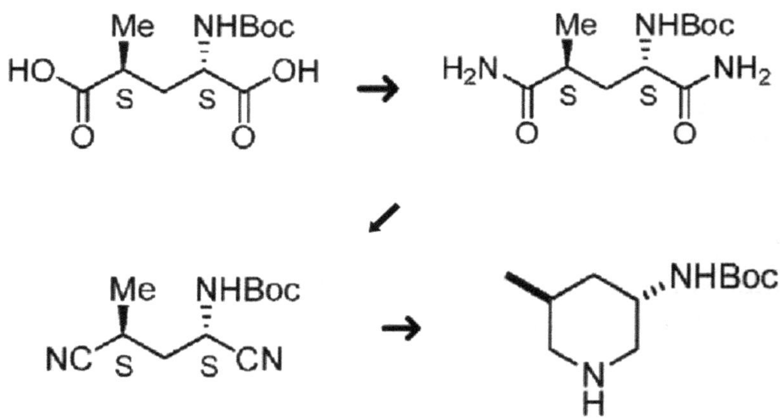

These patents protect:

- Dialdehyde and dinitrile routes from L-glutamic acid
- Intramolecular reductive amination
- Stereochemical control of the 3S,5S configuration
- Oxalate-salt purification
- Downstream coupling to the quinolone core

This became the fourth moat: control of the stereoselective chemistry to the 3S,5S-piperidine side chain.

V. The 2022 API-Purity Patents: Closing the Final Gate

The final moat in Nemonoxacin's manufacturing architecture emerged with the 2022–2024 API-purity patents - US 12,005,059 and CN 114437026A - which protect the quality attributes of the drug substance itself.

US 12,005,059 B2
Title: Nemonoxacin Malate Active Pharmaceutical Ingredient with Low Combination Impurities, and a Preparation Method Thereof

Filed: December 12, 2022
Granted: June 11, 2024
Published (as application US2023/0201189 A1): June 29, 2023
Priority Date: October 26, 2021

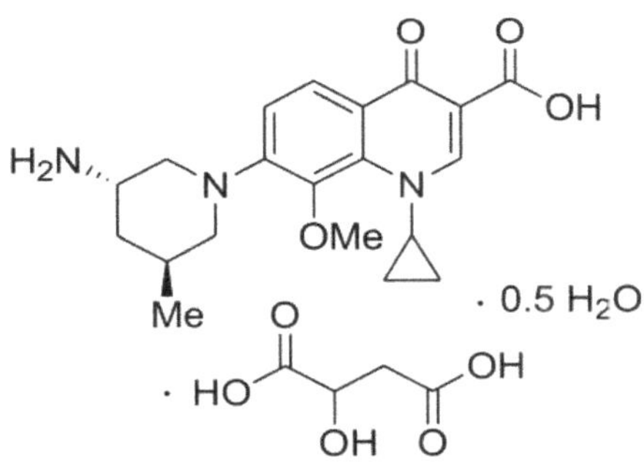

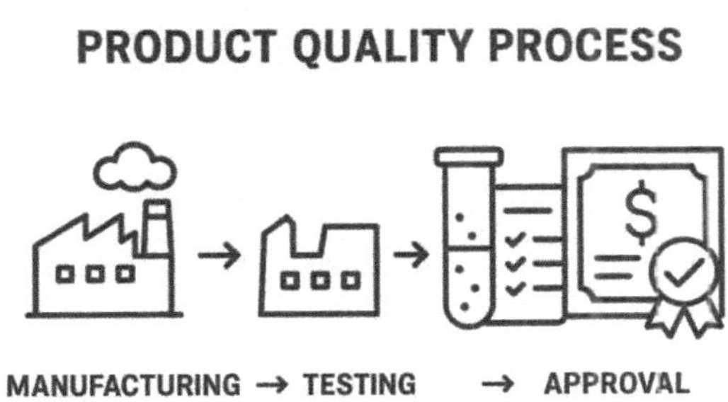

This patent discloses a Nemonoxacin malate API with low combination impurities, produced through a controlled crystallization process using a C1–C3 alcohol/water mixed solvent containing Nemonoxacin free base and D, L-malic acid. Cooling crystallization, followed by solid–liquid separation, washing, and drying, yields an API with significantly reduced impurity levels.

CN 114437026 A
Title: 一种低合成杂质的奈莫沙星苹果酸盐原料药及其制备方法
(Nemonoxacin Malate Active Pharmaceutical Ingredient with Low Combination Impurities, and a Preparation Method Thereof)

Note: This is the Chinese counterpart to US 12,005,059 B2.
Filed: October 26, 2021
Published: May 6, 2022

The Chinese counterpart protects a low-composition-impurity Nemonoxacin malate bulk drug and its preparation method. It uses the same solvent system and crystallization strategy to achieve a high-purity malate hemihydrate form.

Why these patents matter

Together, these filings secure:

- Control of impurity profiles
- Control of crystallization conditions
- Control of solvent systems and cooling parameters
- Control of the final malate hemihydrate form
- Control of regulatory-grade purity specifications

They extend the manufacturing moat into the 2040s, long after the original composition-of-matter patent expired.

Strategic impact

These patents do not merely refine the API - they define the only commercially viable route to a regulatory-acceptable Nemonoxacin malate. Any generic manufacturer must either:

1. Reproduce this impurity-controlled crystallization process (blocked by the patents), or
2. Invent an entirely new purification strategy (highly unlikely without infringing).

Thus, US12005059 and CN114437026A complete the fifth moat: control of the final API quality.

Integrating the Layers: A Protected End-to-End Route

By the time Nemonoxacin entered late-stage development, the manufacturing route was protected at every stage:

1. **Quinolone core intermediates**
• US6,803,469B2 / CN100406443C

2. **Chiral diol precursor (hydride reduction)**
• US7,528,264B2 / CN101045695B

3. **Boron-chelate coupling**
• US7,456,279B2 / CN101045724B

4. **Stereoselective piperidine construction**
• CN102093260B / TWI386395B / WO2010077798

5. **Final API purification (2022 patents)**
• US12005059 and CN114437026A

This is what a manufacturing fortress looks like:

multiple patent families, each guarding a different gate, but all aligned to protect a single commercial route.

The Strategic Role of Manufacturing Patents

Manufacturing patents:

- Block generics through practical necessity
- Extend exclusivity beyond composition-of-matter
- Ensure global supply chain integrity
- Provide leverage in licensing and partnerships

For Nemonoxacin, they transformed a vulnerable molecule into a multi-decade protected asset.

Conclusion - Manufacturing as a Strategic Weapon

The manufacturing layer is where chemistry becomes strategy.
For Nemonoxacin, it was created:

- A protected core
- A protected activated intermediate
- A protected coupling method
- A protected stereochemical side chain
- A protected final API

This is how a drug survives beyond its original patent—
not through a single invention, but through a coordinated architecture of manufacturing IP.

PART III

Regulatory Navigation

Four systems, four cultures, one molecule – and the discipline required to move between them.

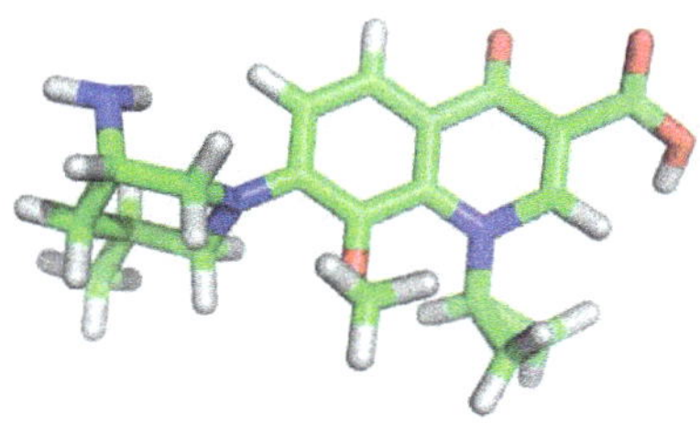

Chapter 9.

The First Regulatory Fork in the Road

The first true divergence in Nemonoxacin's journey emerged not from chemistry or microbiology, but from regulation. A single molecule - PG-873870 - was about to be interpreted by four different regulatory systems, each with its own logic, expectations, and developmental philosophy. This was the moment when the project stopped being purely scientific and became unavoidably geopolitical.

Up to this point, the molecule had lived in a universal language: MIC values, PK curves, toxicology margins. But once it stepped into the regulatory arena, it had to acquire multiple identities. The same data would be read differently by the U.S. FDA, China's NMPA, Taiwan's TFDA, and Russia's Ministry of Health. The first fork in the road was not a choice of direction - it was the realization that there would be no single road at all.

P&G's First Step: The Original U.S. IND

The regulatory journey began in Cincinnati.
Before TaiGen ever touched the molecule, Procter & Gamble Pharmaceuticals submitted the first U.S. IND to the FDA. This IND (IND#68,976) authorized Phase Ia - the first-in-human, single-ascending-dose study.

P&G's rationale was straightforward:

- The U.S. FDA remained the global gold standard for first-in-human safety evaluation.
- A U.S. IND would establish a credible, internationally recognized foundation.
- Early human PK, safety, and tolerability data would be essential for any future global development.

This IND created the molecule's first regulatory identity:

PG-873870 is a first-in-class non-fluorinated quinolone requiring rigorous, stepwise evaluation.

But P&G's strategic priorities shifted. Anti-infectives were no longer a core focus. And so, after Phase Ia, the molecule's regulatory future passed to TaiGen.

TaiGen's First Major Decision: File a New U.S. IND

When TaiGen licensed the molecule in 2004, it inherited P&G's scientific data - but not its regulatory position. P&G's original IND had carried the molecule only through Phase Ia. Once the asset was transferred, the regulatory sponsorship did not.

1. **TaiGen submitted its own U.S. IND (IND#72,088) on April 13, 2005.**

This was not a procedural formality. It was a declaration of ownership - the moment TaiGen assumed full responsibility for the molecule's future in the United States.

2. **Why TaiGen filed a new IND**

- TaiGen needed direct regulatory control over all subsequent clinical development.
- The company was introducing new CMC, new manufacturing sites, and new formulations, none of which could be managed under P&G's IND.
- The FDA required that the active sponsor - the company actually conducting Phase Ib (the first-in-human, multiple-ascending-dose study) and Phase II studies - hold the IND.
- TaiGen's planned Phase Ib and Phase II designs diverged from P&G's original clinical roadmap.

3. **The IND became TaiGen's first regulatory identity.**

With IND#72,088, the molecule transformed from:
PG-873870 under P&G's first-in-human program →
Nemonoxacin under TaiGen's global development leadership.

This decision set the stage for the next, more complex fork in the road: navigating the fundamentally different regulatory philosophies of the United States, China, and - critically - Taiwan.

The U.S.–China Regulatory Divide: Two Systems, Two Definitions

The most consequential divergence came from a simple truth:
The U.S. FDA and China's NMPA did not share the same definitions of Phase I, Phase II, or Phase III.

In the United States (FDA):

- Phase I focuses on safety and PK in healthy volunteers.
- Phase II evaluates dose-response and preliminary efficacy.
- Phase III confirms efficacy and safety in large populations.

In China (then SFDA/CFDA, now NMPA):

- A Class 1.1 new drug required a complete, end-to-end development program within China.
- Local Phase I, Phase II, and Phase III data were expected.
- Imported foreign Phase I data were not automatically accepted.
- The regulatory culture emphasized completeness and domestic validation.

This meant that TaiGen could not simply "port" the U.S. IND into China.

The molecule had to begin again.

TaiGen's China IND: A Full Restart from Phase I → NDA

TaiGen submitted a China IND that initiated:

- China Phase I (oral and IV)
- China Phase II (oral and IV)
- China Phase III (oral and IV)

- Leading ultimately to China NDA approvals for both oral capsules and IV injection

This was not duplication - it was a necessity.

The rationale:

- China's Class 1.1 pathway required a full domestic clinical package.
- China represented the largest future market for Nemonoxacin.
- Local PK, safety, and efficacy data were essential for regulatory acceptance.
- China's hospital bidding and reimbursement systems depended on local clinical evidence.
- The IV formulation, in particular, needed China-specific CMC and clinical validation.

Thus, the molecule acquired its third regulatory identity:
Nemonoxacin is a China Class 1.1 new drug with a complete, locally generated clinical dossier.

This identity would later become the foundation for commercialization in China.

Taiwan: The Fourth Regulatory Identity - A Cross-Strait Clinical Bridge

Taiwan's role in Nemonoxacin's development was unique.
It was neither a full restart (as in China) nor a simple continuation (as in the U.S.).

Instead, Taiwan became a regulatory bridge - a hybrid model that blended:

- China's requirement for local participation
- U.S.-style scientific rigor
- Taiwan's own regulatory independence under the TFDA

Taiwan's TFDA sits between the U.S. and China in regulatory culture

System	Philosophy	Implication for Nemonoxacin
U.S. FDA	Science-driven, modular, flexible	Accepts data if scientifically valid
China NMPA	Domestic completeness, local validation	Requires a full clinical program
Taiwan TFDA	Hybrid: scientific rigor + local participation	Accepts multinational trials with Taiwan sites

1. **TFDA Approval for Participation in China's Phase III Oral Study**

   In January 2010, the Taiwan Food and Drug Administration (TFDA) approved the inclusion of Taiwan clinical sites into China's Phase III oral multicenter trial.

2. **TFDA Approvals for China's Phase II and Phase III IV Studies**

   In 2012, TFDA approved Taiwan's participation in China's Phase II IV multicenter clinical trial for Nemonoxacin IV multicenter trial.

   In 2017, TFDA approved Taiwan's inclusion in China's Phase III IV multicenter trial for Nemonoxacin IV multicenter trial.

Thus, Taiwan created a fourth regulatory identity:

Nemonoxacin is a cross-strait, TFDA-recognized drug supported by local Phase III oral and local Phase II/Phase III IV participation. This identity later enabled Taiwan's own regulatory review and approval pathway.

The R-Pharm Partnership and the Russian IND

The fourth major regulatory pathway emerged after TaiGen signed the exclusive licensing agreement with R-Pharm in 2014.

Russia's Ministry of Health required:

- A Russian IND
- A Phase III bridging study conducted under Russian GCP
- Local confirmatory evidence to support registration

The rationale for the Russian IND was distinct:

- Russia did not require a full end-to-end development program.
- Instead, it required a bridging study to confirm that the global data applied to the Russian population.
- The Russian regulatory culture emphasized procedural completeness and domestic clinical verification.

Thus, the molecule gained its fifth regulatory identity:
Nemonoxacin is a globally developed drug requiring Russian confirmatory evidence for local approval.

This pathway ultimately led to Russian marketing authorization in 2022.

Four Systems, Four Cultures, One Molecule

By the time Nemonoxacin reached its first global approvals, it had lived four different regulatory lives:

Region	Regulatory Pathway	Sponsor	Clinical Scope
United States	US IND (P&G → TaiGen)	US IND (P&G Ia → TaiGen Ib-II)	Early human safety, PK, dosing-finding
China	China IND (Class 1.1)	TaiGen	Full Phase I → Phase III → NDA (oral + IV)
Taiwan	TFDA approval for participation in China Phase III oral and	TaiGen	Local Phase III oral and Phase II/Phase III IV sites; basis for

	Phase II/Phase III IV		Taiwan approvals
Russia	Russian IND	R-Pharm (under TaiGen license)	Phase III bridging study

The following table presents a consolidated visual timeline capturing all major regulatory submissions and approvals across the United States, China, Taiwan, and Russia throughout the development of Nemonoxacin.

GLOBAL REGULATORY TIMELINE PG-873870 → NEMONOXACIN (1998-2022)	
1998-2004	Procter & Gamble (R&G) • Preclinical discovery and development of PG-873870
2004	P&G → U.S. FDA • Original U.S. IND submitted • Authorization for Phase Ia (first-in-human SAD)
Dec 2004	P&G licenses PG-873870 to TaiGen • Scientific package transferred • Regulatory sponsorship does NOT transfer
UNITED STATES REGULATORY PATHWAY	
Apr 2005	TaiGen submits NEW U.S. IND (IND#72,088) • Establishes TaiGen as the NEW regulatory sponsor • Enables Phase Ib → Phase II development
CHINA REGULATORY PATHWAY (NMPA)	
Sept 2006 2016 2021	TaiGen submits Class 1.1 New Drug to the China FDA • China Phase I (oral + IV) • China Phase II (oral + IV) • China Phase III (oral + IV) China NDA submissions and approvals • Oral capsules approved • IV injection approved

TAIWAN REGULATORY CROSS-STRAIT PATHWAY (TFDA)	
2010 2012 2014 2020	TaiGen received TFDA approval for Taiwan sites in the China Phase III oral TaiGen received TFDA approval for Taiwan sites in China Phase II/Phase III IV Taiwan NDA submission and approval • Oral capsules approved • IV injection approved
RUSSIA REGULATORY PATHWAY (MoH)	
2014 2015-2016 2022	TaiGen signs exclusive licensing agreement with R-Pharm Russian IND submitted • Russian Phase III bridging study initiated Russian marketing authorization granted

The molecule was the same.

The science was the same.

But the regulatory identities were different - because the systems were different.

This was the first regulatory fork in the road, and it shaped everything that followed.

Why This Fork Matters

This chapter marks the moment TaiGen realized that global drug development is not a linear path. It is a branching network of regulatory expectations, cultural interpretations, and strategic decisions.

The first fork taught the team:

- A molecule must be translated, not merely submitted.
- Regulatory systems reflect national priorities and cultural logic.
- A global program requires multiple identities, not one.
- Strategic sequencing is as important as scientific excellence.
- The sponsor must adapt - the molecule cannot.

From this point forward, Nemonoxacin's journey would be defined by its ability to navigate these parallel systems without losing coherence, integrity, or momentum.

The first fork was not an obstacle.

It was the beginning of global identity.

Chapter 10.

Navigating Four Systems at Once

How one molecule required four regulatory languages - and four CMC dialects - to move forward.

The first regulatory fork taught TaiGen that Nemonoxacin would not travel on a single road. But the deeper challenge - the one that defined the next decade - was learning to move through four regulatory systems simultaneously, each with its own scientific expectations, cultural logic, and CMC requirements.

The molecule was the same.

The science was the same.

But the regulatory chemistry was not.

CMC - Chemistry, Manufacturing, and Controls - became the quiet backbone of global navigation. It was the part of the program that could never fail, never drift, never contradict itself. And yet, it had to be expressed differently in each system.

Parallel development meant parallel CMC identities.

Four Systems, Four CMC Expectations

Each regulatory authority interpreted the molecule through its own manufacturing, quality, and process-control lens. TaiGen had to maintain a single scientific truth while adapting the CMC narrative to four distinct frameworks.

1. United States: Modular, Data-Driven, and Comparability-Focused

Under U.S. IND#72,088, the FDA expected:

- Clear definition of regulatory starting materials (RSMs) - MAP and FABE - and their control strategies.
- GMP manufacturing consistency across multiple sites (P&G → AMRI → UPM).
- Stability data demonstrating long-term control (36-month stability at 25°C/60% RH).
- CMC amendments aligned with evolving clinical phases (Phase Ib → Phase II).
- Comparability packages when API manufacturing moved from P&G to AMRI.

The U.S. system treated CMC as a living document. Every change - new GMP batch, new impurity profile, new stability data - required transparent justification. This modularity allowed flexibility, but it also demanded discipline.

The U.S. CMC identity of Nemonoxacin was:

A well-characterized, GMP-controlled drug substance and capsule product with traceable lineage from P&G's Norwich facility to AMRI's large-scale API and UPM's clinical drug product manufacturing.

2. China: Domestic Completeness and End-to-End CMC Validation

China's Class 1.1 pathway required a full domestic CMC ecosystem:

- Domestic API manufacturing at Wisdom Pharma (Haimen, Jiangsu).
- Domestic analytical validation at China Pharmaceutical University.
- Domestic capsule manufacturing at Hua-Yu (WuXi).
- Multiple GMP API campaigns (21.5 kg → 42 kg → 3 × 40 kg validation batches).
- Stability studies supporting long-term storage (48-month stability at 25°C/60% RH).
- API process optimization and scale-up (dinitrile route improvements for MAP).

- NDA-ready validation batches of API and drug product produced at Xinchang Pharmaceutical Factory (ZMC).

China's regulatory culture required that the molecule be born again within its borders - not only clinically, but chemically.

The China CMC identity of Nemonoxacin was:

A domestically manufactured Class 1.1 new drug with complete, China-generated API, analytical, and drug-product data supporting Phase I → III → NDA.

3. Taiwan: Cross-Strait CMC Alignment with Independent TFDA Review

Taiwan's TFDA required a hybrid approach:

- CMC alignment with China's manufacturing data, since Taiwan sites participated in China's Phase III oral and Phase II/III IV trials.
- Independent TFDA review of API and capsule specifications.
- Local drug-product manufacturing for Taiwan NDA and commercialization (Lotus Pharma, Nangkuang Pharma).
- Use of China-validated API (e.g., 60 kg batches from Wisdom's 2012 campaign).
- Cross-strait comparability to ensure Taiwan's clinical data were scientifically interchangeable with China's.

Taiwan did not require a full domestic CMC rebuild, but it required CMC transparency, traceability, and equivalence.

The Taiwan CMC identity of Nemonoxacin was:

A cross-strait drug product whose API and manufacturing lineage were China-validated but Taiwan-reviewed, enabling TFDA approval based on shared clinical and CMC foundations.

4. Russia: Dossier-Driven CMC Translation and Local Verification

Russia's Ministry of Health required:

- A complete CMC dossier mapping global data into the Russian regulatory structure.
- Local confirmatory evidence through a Phase III bridging study.
- Clear traceability of API manufacturing (P&G → AMRI → Wisdom → ZMC).
- Demonstration that global GMP processes met Russian standards.
- Stability, impurity, and process-control data presented in Russian format.

Russia did not require domestic manufacturing, but it required domestic interpretability — a full translation of global CMC logic into Russian regulatory language.

The Russian CMC identity of Nemonoxacin was:

A globally manufactured drug substance and product whose quality, stability, and process controls were verified through a Russian bridging study and dossier review.

CMC as the Hidden Architecture of Parallel Navigation

While clinical teams managed protocols, enrollment, and data, the CMC teams carried the structural burden of global coherence.

They had to ensure:

- One molecule, four dossiers
- One synthetic route, multiple GMP campaigns
- One impurity profile, multiple analytical standards
- One stability narrative, multiple regulatory interpretations
- One global supply chain, multiple local requirements

CMC became the discipline that held the entire global program together.

Without CMC coherence, the four regulatory identities would have fractured into four different molecules.

CMC Architecture Across Four Regulatory Systems

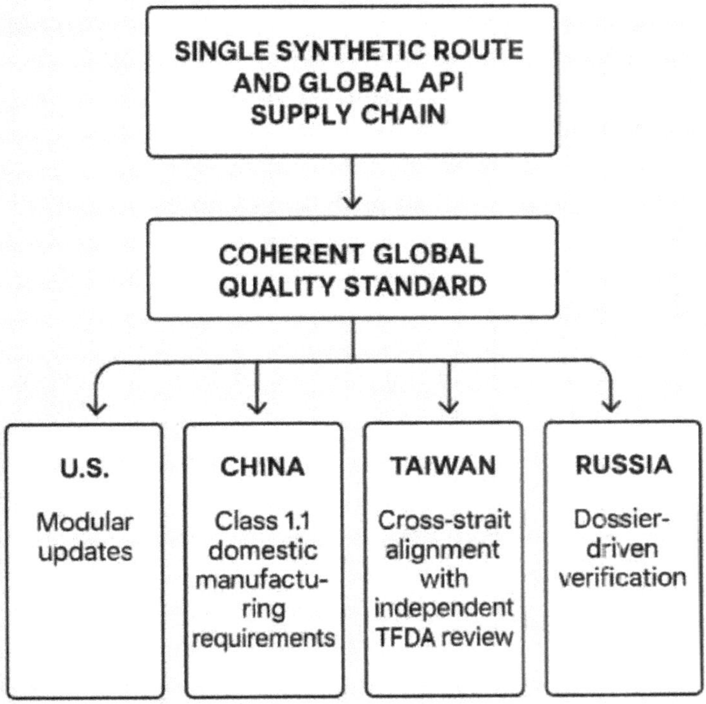

This diagram maps how a single synthetic route and global API supply chain were translated into four distinct CMC identities—U.S. modular updates, China's Class 1.1 domestic manufacturing requirements, Taiwan's cross-strait alignment with independent TFDA review, and Russia's dossier-driven verification—while preserving one coherent global quality standard.

The Strategic Burden of Being First – Chemically

Nemonoxacin was not only first-in-class clinically. It was first-in-class chemically:

- A non-fluorinated quinolone
- A novel D,L-malate hemihydrate salt (TG-875649)

- A molecule with no prior regulatory precedent
- A drug requiring new analytical methods, new impurity controls, and new stability models

Every regulatory system had to be educated - not only about the clinical program, but about the chemistry itself.

CMC was not background work.

It was the language through which each system understood the molecule.

Why CMC Integration Mattered

CMC was the only part of the program that touched every system equally. It was the backbone of:

- IND submissions
- CTA approvals
- NDA filings
- GMP inspections
- Technology transfers
- Commercial readiness

CMC was also the only domain where failure in one system could jeopardize all others.

Parallel navigation required:

- U.S. modularity
- China completeness
- Taiwan cross-strait alignment
- Russia dossier translation

And CMC had to satisfy all four simultaneously.

The Lesson of Chapter 10

If Chapter 9 reveals the first regulatory fork, Chapter 10 reveals the deeper truth:

Global drug development is not only clinical navigation - it is CMC orchestration.

TaiGen succeeded not because it chose the right path, but because it learned to sustain four paths at once, chemically and clinically, without losing the molecule's identity.

Nemonoxacin survived four systems because its CMC foundation was strong enough to support four regulatory cultures simultaneously.

This was the discipline that made global development possible.

Chapter 11.

Aligning Patents with Regulatory Exclusivity

Nemonoxacin's global development journey demonstrates a strategic alignment between patent protection and regulatory exclusivity across multiple jurisdictions. This chapter integrates TaiGen's acquisition of worldwide patent rights - initially transferred from Procter & Gamble Pharmaceuticals (P&GP) and later expanded through TaiGen's own inventions - with the regulatory pathways in the United States, China, Taiwan, and Russia.

The combination of composition-of-matter patents, new TaiGen-invented patents, the latest 2022 API-Purity patents, and regulatory exclusivity windows now extends meaningful protection for Nemonoxacin into the 2040s, ensuring long-term commercial value and lifecycle sustainability.

TaiGen's Global Patent Position as the Foundation of Exclusivity

TaiGen's regulatory strategy was only possible because of its comprehensive ownership of the Nemonoxacin patent estate, which unfolded in three major phases:

1. Transfer of P&G's Global Patent Portfolio (2005)

In early 2005, TaiGen received all worldwide patents and patent applications related to Nemonoxacin from P&GP.

This included:

- Composition-of-matter patents (e.g., US 6,329,391)
- Process patents
- Polymorph patents
- Intermediate and synthetic-route patents

These patents were granted across 37 countries, forming the backbone of global exclusivity.

2. Consolidation After Warner Chilcott Acquisition (2009–2011)

When Warner Chilcott acquired P&G's pharmaceutical division in 2009, TaiGen renegotiated and retained all Asian rights.

In 2011, TaiGen secured full global development rights, enabling:

- Unified CMC strategy
- Global regulatory submissions
- Freedom to file new patents

3. New Patents Invented by TaiGen (2008–2013)

TaiGen expanded exclusivity through five new patent families, including:

- Parenteral formulation (CN101361739B)
- Antibiotic-resistant infection treatment
- Pneumonia treatment
- New synthetic routes
- Stereoselective piperidine synthesis

These patents extended protection well beyond the original P&G estate, especially in China and Taiwan.

4. China Patents Transfer to ZMC (2012–2021)

For China's commercialization, TaiGen transferred 13 Chinese patents to Zhejiang Medicine Co. (ZMC).

This transfer later enabled ZMC to become the Marketing Authorization Holder (MAH) under China's 2020 regulatory reforms.

Together, these patent layers enabled TaiGen to synchronize IP protection with regulatory exclusivity windows in every jurisdiction.

United States Strategy: Patent Layering and Qualified Infectious Disease Product (QIDP) Designation

Patent Protection

TaiGen inherited and expanded the U.S. patent estate from P&G, including:

- Composition-of-matter patents
- Salt-form patents for TG-875649
- Process and intermediate patents

TaiGen's later filings (e.g., pneumonia-treatment patents) provided additional lifecycle extension.

Regulatory Exclusivity

Under Investigational New Drug (IND) application number 72,088, TaiGen secured:

- Qualified Infectious Disease Product (QIDP) designation
- Fast Track designation for:
- Community-acquired bacterial pneumonia (CABP)
- Acute bacterial skin and skin structure infections (ABSSSI)

These designations enabled:

- 5-year exclusivity extension under the Generating Antibiotic Incentives Now (GAIN) Act
- Priority review and accelerated development timelines

CMC Identity

Modular IND updates allowed integration of China Phase II/III data and manufacturing validations.

TaiGen's full patent ownership enabled consistent global CMC control, a prerequisite for cross-referenced data packages.

China Strategy: Class 1.1 Registration and Domestic Manufacturing

Patent Protection

China filings mirrored the U.S. estate but added:

- Polymorph patents (e.g., CN101045725B)
- Process patents
- Parenteral formulation patents (CN101361739B)

In 2012, TaiGen transferred all China Nemonoxacin patents to ZMC to support local commercialization and later MAH designation.

Regulatory Exclusivity

Nemonoxacin was classified as a Class 1.1 new chemical drug, granting:

- 6-year data exclusivity
- Eligibility for priority review
- Protection reinforced by local manufacturing requirements

CMC Identity

China's dossier emphasized:

- Domestic API production (Wisdom → ZMC)
- Domestic drug product manufacturing (Hua-Yu → ZMC)
- Analytical support (China Pharmaceutical University → ZMC)
- Patent ownership transfer enabled ZMC to meet China's MAH regulatory reforms in 2020.

Taiwan Strategy: Cross-Strait Clinical Integration with Independent Review

Patent Protection

Taiwan filings were synchronized with the global estate, including TaiGen's own patents.

Taiwan's patent protection was essential for:

- Local manufacturing (Lotus, Nangkuang)
- Regional commercialization (ASEAN, Russia supply)

Regulatory Exclusivity

The Taiwan Food and Drug Administration (TFDA) approved Taiwan's participation in:

- China's Phase III oral trial
- China's Phase II/III intravenous trials

This arrangement:

- Enabled dual-site data integration
- Preserved Taiwan's independent regulatory pathway

CMC Identity

Oral capsules were manufactured by Lotus Pharmaceutical, and intravenous injection was manufactured by Nangkuang Pharmaceutical. Both are aligned with China's validated API batches.

Russia Strategy: Dossier-Driven Verification

Patent Protection

Russia relied on translated versions of TaiGen's global patent portfolio, including:

- Composition-of-matter
- Process
- Formulation patents

These patents provided enforceable exclusivity in the absence of formal data-exclusivity statutes.

Regulatory Exclusivity

The Ministry of Health (Minzdrav) granted approval based on:

- Full dossier submission (China Phase I–III + Taiwan validations)
- Local pharmacovigilance and post-marketing commitments

CMC Identity

Russia accepted the global synthetic route and API supply chain.

And GMP compliance at Nangkuang (Taiwan) was verified through pre-approval inspection.

Unified Quality Standard Across Jurisdictions

Despite jurisdictional differences, TaiGen maintained a single global CMC identity, enabled by its patent ownership and control of the synthetic route.

All four CMC identities - United States, China, Taiwan, and Russia - were harmonized through shared regulatory starting materials:

- MAP (methyl-aminopyridine intermediate)
- FABE (fluoro-aminobutyric ester intermediate)
- Consistent GMP manufacturing protocols
- Stability data supporting long-term shelf life
- Cross-referenced analytical and clinical data packages

Patent ownership ensured that no jurisdiction diverged in synthetic route, impurity profile, or analytical standards.

Strategic Takeaways

- Patent protection and regulatory exclusivity are mutually reinforcing tools for lifecycle management.
- TaiGen's acquisition of worldwide patent rights enabled global CMC harmonization, cross-referenced clinical data, and synchronized regulatory submissions.

- Jurisdiction-specific tailoring of CMC dossiers enabled local compliance without fragmenting global quality.
- Cross-border clinical integration - such as China–Taiwan collaboration - enhanced regulatory credibility and market access.
- Early alignment of patent filings with regulatory strategy maximized exclusivity duration and commercial value.
- Strategic patent transfers (e.g., to ZMC) enabled compliance with evolving regulatory frameworks such as China's MAH system.

PART IV

Commercialization

This is where the molecule leaves the lab and enters the world.

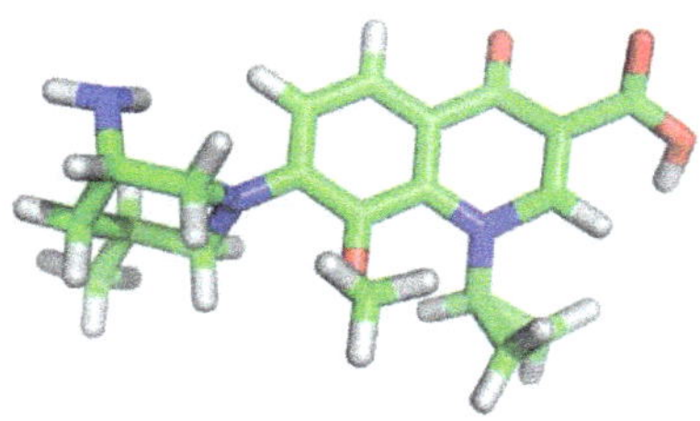

Chapter 12.

A Molecule Meets the Market

When a drug finally reaches the market, the scientific journey that began with a single molecular idea collides with the realities of medicine, economics, and human need.

For Nemonoxacin, this moment was not a single event but a sequence of carefully orchestrated transitions - each one transforming the molecule from a promising clinical candidate into a therapeutic agent trusted by physicians and relied upon by patients. After years of discovery, development, regulatory negotiation, and manufacturing refinement, Nemonoxacin was ready to meet the world.

From Clinical Data to Commercial Identity

By the time the first approvals arrived, Nemonoxacin had already accumulated a dossier of evidence: its broad-spectrum activity, its potency against drug-resistant pathogens, its favorable safety profile, and its dual oral–intravenous flexibility. Yet none of these attributes alone guaranteed commercial success. A drug must not only work, but it must also be manufacturable, stable, transportable, prescribable, reimbursable, and recognizable.

The transition from “TG-873870” to “Nemonoxacin,” and ultimately to Taigexyn®, marked the beginning of its commercial identity. The molecule that once existed only in laboratory notebooks and regulatory submissions now had a name that physicians could write on prescriptions and pharmacists could place on shelves. The brand carried the weight of Taiwan’s first self-developed new chemical entity, a milestone that resonated far beyond the walls of TaiGen.

The First Launch: Taiwan’s Milestone (2014 Approval; 2015 Launch)

Taiwan granted marketing approval for the 250-mg oral capsule in March 2014, marking the first regulatory authorization for Nemonoxacin anywhere in the world. Commercial launch followed in mid-2015, transforming the molecule from a scientific achievement into a national symbol.

For the first time, a Taiwanese company had shepherded a new chemical entity from discovery to market authorization. The approval validated not only the science behind Nemonoxacin but also the infrastructure, discipline, and ambition of Taiwan's biotechnology sector.

The commercial rollout required coordination across manufacturing, distribution, medical affairs, and marketing. Lotus Pharmaceutical produced the first GMP commercial batches, each capsule carrying the light-blue imprint of a drug that symbolized a decade of effort. Holding Pharma managed distribution, ensuring that Taigexyn® reached hospitals, clinics, and pharmacies across the island.

Physicians responded with curiosity and cautious optimism. An antibiotic active against quinolone-resistant Streptococcus pneumoniae and MRSA, yet without the fluorine atom associated with many quinolone toxicities, represented a rare addition to the antimicrobial armamentarium. Early clinical use confirmed what the trials had suggested: Nemonoxacin filled a therapeutic gap.

Cross-Strait Momentum: China Joins the Market (2016 Approval; 2017 Launch)

China's National Medical Products Administration (NMPA) approved the oral capsule in June 2016, marking the second major commercial milestone. Commercial launch began in 2017, supported by the scale and reach of China's hospital system.

Zhejiang Medicine Co. Ltd. (ZMC), TaiGen's commercial partner, assumed responsibility for manufacturing and distribution. Their Xinchang facility produced the GMP batches that would supply hospitals across China. The collaboration demonstrated a rare cross-strait synergy: Taiwanese innovation paired with Chinese industrial capacity.

For clinicians in China, Taigexyn® offered a new option for community-acquired pneumonia at a time when antimicrobial resistance was accelerating. Its low propensity for resistance development, demonstrated in both laboratory and clinical settings, became a key differentiator in a crowded therapeutic landscape.

The Intravenous Era: Expanding Clinical Reach (Taiwan 2020; China 2021)

The introduction of the intravenous formulation marked a turning point. Oral antibiotics serve outpatients and mild cases; intravenous formulations serve the critically ill. With the 500 mg/250 mL LVP soft bag, Nemonoxacin entered emergency rooms, intensive care units, and inpatient wards.

- Taiwan approved the IV formulation in October 2020.
- China approved the IV formulation in June 2021.

Hospitals now had the flexibility to initiate therapy intravenously and transition patients to oral capsules - a continuity of care that strengthened Nemonoxacin's clinical utility.

The IV formulation also signaled the maturation of TaiGen's CMC capabilities. Large-volume parenterals demand stringent sterility, stability, and packaging controls. The successful validation of manufacturing sites in Taiwan and China demonstrated that the molecule could be produced reliably at scale.

Global Expansion: Russia and Beyond (Russia Approval 2022)

The Russian Ministry of Health approved Nemonoxacin in 2022, secured through TaiGen's partnership with R-Pharm. The Phase III trial conducted across Russia provided local clinical evidence, reinforcing the drug's credibility among regional physicians.

With this approval, Taigexyn® became a multinational brand, available in oral and intravenous forms across Asia and Eastern Europe.

Additional licensing agreements opened pathways into Latin America, Southeast Asia, and English-speaking markets.

Each new territory required adaptation - regulatory dossiers tailored to local requirements, manufacturing audits, pharmacovigilance systems, and market education. Yet the core message remained constant: Nemonoxacin was a modern antibiotic designed for an era of rising resistance.

A Molecule in the Hands of Physicians

Once a drug reaches the market, its fate lies not in laboratories or boardrooms but in the decisions of physicians treating real patients. Reports began to emerge from hospitals:

- elderly patients with community-acquired pneumonia responding rapidly to therapy
- cases of quinolone-resistant S. pneumoniae successfully treated
- clinicians appreciating the once-daily dosing and oral–IV switch flexibility

These stories, though anecdotal, represented the true measure of success. A molecule that began as PG-873870 in a P&G laboratory was now saving lives in Taiwan, China, Russia, and beyond.

The Market as the Final Test

Commercialization is often described as the "last mile" of drug development, but in reality, it is a new beginning. The market tests a drug in ways no clinical trial can fully anticipate: prescribing habits, reimbursement pressures, supply chain resilience, competition, and the unpredictable dynamics of antimicrobial stewardship.

For Nemonoxacin, the market validated its scientific promise. Physicians adopted it, regulators endorsed it, and manufacturers produced it at scale. The molecule had crossed the threshold from experimental compound to therapeutic agent.

A Legacy Still Unfolding

As Nemonoxacin continues to expand into new indications and territories, its story remains unfinished. Phase IV studies, real-world evidence, and ongoing clinical trials in CAP, UTI, and COPD exacerbations will shape its future role in global medicine.

But one milestone is already secure: Nemonoxacin met the market—and the market welcomed it.

Chapter 13.

The First Real-World Signals

When a drug enters the market, it steps out of the controlled universe of clinical trials and into the unfiltered complexity of real medicine. No protocol can fully anticipate how physicians will prescribe, how patients will respond, or how healthcare systems will absorb a new therapeutic option. For Nemonoxacin, the first months and years after launch became a second proving ground - one defined not by statistical endpoints but by human variability, clinical pragmatism, and the quiet vigilance of post-marketing surveillance.

In Taiwan and China, this transition unfolded alongside a series of regulatory and market-access milestones - IV approvals, reimbursement decisions, and commercial realignments - that shaped how the drug entered clinical practice. These events did not sit outside the real-world story; they were part of it, influencing who received the drug, how hospitals adopted it, and how physicians incorporated it into their therapeutic routines.

From Trial Populations to Real Patients

Clinical trials are designed to answer specific questions under tightly controlled conditions. Real-world practice is not. Patients arrive with comorbidities, polypharmacy, atypical presentations, and social circumstances that no protocol can fully capture. Physicians make decisions under pressure, often empirically, guided by experience as much as by guidelines.

As Taigexyn® entered hospitals and clinics in Taiwan and China - supported by Taiwan's 2020 IV approval and China's 2020 reimbursement listing for the oral formulation - the first real-world signals began to emerge:

- elderly patients with multiple chronic conditions responding more quickly than expected
- cases of quinolone-resistant Streptococcus pneumoniae resolving without escalation

- physicians using the oral–IV switch strategy more aggressively than anticipated
- shorter hospital stays in certain CAP cohorts, hinting at economic benefits

These early observations did not replace clinical trial data, but they added texture - revealing how the molecule behaved in the messy, unpredictable reality of everyday medicine.

Key Post-Launch Events for Nemonoxacin in Taiwan and China

Year	Taiwan	China
2020	• TFDA approval of IV formulation • Expansion of hospital formulary adoption begins	• Oral formulation added to the National Reimbursement Drug List (NRDL)
2021	-	• NMPA approval of IV formulation • Transfer of MAH and commercial rights to Zhejiang Medicine (ZMC)
2022	• NHI reimbursement eligibility for IV formulation	-
On-going	• Continued pharmacovigilance and microbiological surveillance in CAP and the comorbid population • Real-world evidence accumulation	• Post-market safety monitoring under the MAH system • Exploration of broader pneumonia subtypes and pediatric potential

Early Post-Marketing Surveillance: The Quiet Watchfulness

Every new drug enters the market accompanied by a structured pharmacovigilance system. For Nemonoxacin, this system became the backbone of its early real-world life.

Key components included:

- spontaneous adverse event reporting from hospitals and pharmacies
- periodic safety update reports (PSURs) submitted to regulators
- targeted follow-up on specific patient groups, such as the elderly or those with renal impairment

.• ongoing microbiological surveillance to monitor resistance trends

The early data were reassuring. No unexpected safety signals emerged. The adverse events observed - mild gastrointestinal symptoms, transient liver enzyme elevations - mirrored the clinical trial profile. Importantly, the absence of fluoroquinolone-associated toxicities reinforced the value of Nemonoxacin's non-fluorinated design.

As Taiwan prepared for NHI reimbursement of the IV formulation (granted in 2020) and China moved toward IV approval in 2021, pharmacovigilance teams in both markets intensified their monitoring. These regulatory milestones were not administrative footnotes - they expanded the drug's reach, increasing the diversity of patients contributing to the real-world evidence base.

Real-World Evidence vs. Clinical Expectations

Real-world evidence (RWE) often diverges from clinical trial expectations - not because the drug changes, but because the world does.

For Nemonoxacin, several patterns emerged:

1. Broader patient diversity

Physicians prescribed Taigexyn® to patients excluded from trials - those with unstable comorbidities, borderline renal function, or atypical pneumonia presentations. The drug's performance in these groups expanded its clinical persona.

2. Faster-than-expected symptom resolution

Some hospitals reported shorter fever durations and earlier discharge in CAP patients, prompting interest in health-economic analyses.

3. Lower-than-expected resistance emergence

Microbiology labs in Taiwan and China noted stable susceptibility patterns, reinforcing the molecule's low propensity for resistance development.

4. Adoption of the oral–IV switch model

The dual formulation allowed physicians to initiate therapy intravenously and transition to oral dosing earlier than with many comparators. This flexibility became a defining feature of real-world use.

These signals did not rewrite the label, but they shaped how clinicians perceived the drug - its strengths, its nuances, and its place in therapy.

How Regulators Interpreted the Early Data

Regulatory agencies view the post-marketing period as an extension of the approval process. For Nemonoxacin, the early real-world data informed:

- renewal of marketing authorizations
- updates to safety sections of product labels
- refinements to risk-management plans
- consideration of new indications based on emerging evidence

In Taiwan, the absence of serious safety concerns supported the continued expansion of hospital formulary adoption. This period also coincided with TFDA approval of the IV formulation in 2020, followed by NHI reimbursement eligibility in 2022, which accelerated uptake in tertiary hospitals and broadened access across regional medical centers.

In China, early RWE contributed to discussions around broader pneumonia subtypes and potential pediatric development. These clinical signals unfolded alongside major market-access and commercial events:

- 2020 inclusion of the oral formulation in China's national reimbursement list, which dramatically expanded patient access

- 2021 approval of the IV formulation, enabling full inpatient–outpatient coverage
- 2021 transfer of China rights to Zhejiang Medicine, which reshaped the commercial and pharmacovigilance responsibilities under China's MAH system

In Russia, local Phase III data combined with early post-launch experience strengthened confidence among infectious disease specialists.

Regulators were not merely observers - they were active interpreters of the molecule's evolving identity.

Inside the Company: Vigilance, Analytics, and Strategic Adjustment

For TaiGen and its partners, the post-marketing period demanded a new organizational posture. The focus shifted from development to stewardship.

1. Pharmacovigilance teams

Monitored global safety databases, triaged reports, and coordinated with regulators.

2. Medical affairs

Engaged with physicians, collected real-world insights, and supported appropriate use through education and stewardship programs.

3. Commercial analytics

Tracked prescribing patterns, formulary decisions, and regional adoption curves to identify unmet needs and opportunities.

In China, analytics teams closely monitored the impact of reimbursement inclusion and the transition to Zhejiang Medicine as MAH.

In Taiwan, the IV formulation's reimbursement milestone reshaped hospital procurement behavior.

4. Clinical development

Used real-world signals to refine ongoing and future trials in CAP, UTI, and COPD exacerbations.

The company's internal response was not reactive - it was adaptive. Each new data point informed strategy, ensuring that the molecule's real-world life was guided as carefully as its development had been.

A Molecule Finding Its Place in Medicine

The first real-world signals did more than validate Nemonoxacin's clinical promise - they revealed its emerging identity as a therapeutic agent:

- a modern antibiotic suited for an era of rising resistance
- a flexible option for both outpatient and inpatient care
- a molecule whose safety and efficacy translated beyond the confines of trials
- a drug that physicians trusted enough to use in complex, real-world scenarios

The transition from controlled trials to clinical reality is where many drugs falter. Nemonoxacin did not. It adapted, it performed, and it began to carve out a role in the global management of community-acquired infections.

The Beginning of a New Phase

Market entry was not the end of Nemonoxacin's journey - it was the beginning of a new, unpredictable chapter. Real-world evidence would continue to accumulate, resistance patterns would evolve, and new indications would emerge. The molecule's story was no longer written solely by scientists or regulators; it was now shaped by physicians, patients, and the complex ecosystems of healthcare systems around the world.

The first real-world signals were clear:

Nemonoxacin was not just surviving in the market - it was thriving in the hands of clinicians.

Chapter 14.

How a Molecule Performs in the Real World: Subgroups, Comorbidities, and High-Risk Patients

When a molecule enters the market, it does not simply encounter "patients." It encounters variation - age, organ function, comorbidities, pathogen risk, prior drug exposure, and the unpredictable diversity of real-world clinical practice.

Clinical trials can anticipate some of this heterogeneity, but they cannot fully reproduce it. Only after launch does a molecule begin to reveal how it behaves across the full spectrum of human biology.

For Nemonoxacin, this phase of its life generated a surprisingly rich body of evidence. What began as a narrow set of post-marketing observations gradually expanded into a multidimensional map of special populations, each offering a different lens on the molecule's pharmacology, safety, and clinical utility. Much of this is now consolidated in a comprehensive safety and special-population review that integrates Phase II/III, Phase IV, PK studies, observational cohorts, and a five-year post-marketing surveillance program [2].

This chapter synthesizes that landscape.

1. Renal Impairment: When Clearance Becomes the Story

The most rigorous special-population study conducted for Nemonoxacin focused on **severe renal impairment**, a group often underrepresented in trials but central to antimicrobial stewardship. In a single-dose, open-label, parallel-group PK/PD study, 10 patients with severe renal impairment were compared with 10 matched healthy controls after a 0.5-g oral dose of Nemonoxacin [1].

As summarized in the post-market document:

"Renal impairment significantly reduced urinary excretion (23.4% vs. 66.1%). A two-compartment PK model was established. Monte Carlo simulations were used to evaluate target attainment."

The published analysis confirmed that the data were best described by a two-compartment population PK model, with markedly reduced urinary excretion and altered clearance in the severe-impairment group, and used Monte Carlo simulations to propose dose-adjustment strategies in this population [1].

This study became the foundation for regulatory labeling and dose-adjustment recommendations in severe renal impairment, in line with the broader regulatory framework that emphasizes dedicated PK studies in renal dysfunction [3].

In contrast, **mild–moderate renal impairment** (creatinine clearance ≥50 mL/min) did not require dose adjustment. The systematic safety review, which included special-population PK data, concluded that exposure remained within the therapeutic window and that standard dosing was appropriate in this group [2].

2. Elderly patients: Stability across age

Elderly patients represent a critical real-world subgroup, often carrying multiple comorbidities and polypharmacy risks. The systematic review of oral Nemonoxacin safety integrated:

- Three Phase II/III comparator trials
- One Phase IV study
- Two special-population PK studies
- Four observational studies
- A five-year post-marketing surveillance project (>257,000 patients (Frontiers))

The document captures the key conclusion:

"Across ~1,450 clinical trial patients and >257,000 postmarketing patients, Nemonoxacin was generally well tolerated. No dose adjustment required in elderly patients, supported by Phase IV data."

The review explicitly notes that PK data and Phase IV outcomes support **no dose adjustment in elderly patients**, and that the safety profile is broadly comparable to levofloxacin but without the characteristic fluoroquinolone-class toxicities that have constrained that class in recent years [2,5].

3. Hepatic impairment: A quiet but important signal

Although no dedicated **severe hepatic-impairment** trial has been reported, patients with **mild–moderate hepatic impairment** were included in the special-population PK datasets summarized in the systematic review [2,5].

As the document states:

"No clinically meaningful PK changes reported. No dose adjustment recommended for mild–moderate hepatic impairment. No dedicated severe hepatic impairment study published."

The review concludes that Nemonoxacin demonstrates a stable safety profile in mild–moderate hepatic impairment, with no need for dose adjustment - an important practical consideration in regions with high burdens of chronic liver disease [2].

3. Diabetes: A Contrast with Fluoroquinolones

Fluoroquinolones carry well-recognized risks of dysglycemia. In contrast, Nemonoxacin's real-world data from post-marketing surveillance in China and Taiwan and Phase IV CAP cohorts did **not** reveal a dysglycemia signal.

The document summarizes:

"No signal for dysglycemia (unlike fluoroquinolones). Clinical cure rates are comparable to nondiabetic patients. No PK interaction with glucose-lowering agents reported."

These findings, drawn from the integrated safety and post-marketing datasets, position Nemonoxacin as a more metabolically neutral option in diabetic patients compared with traditional fluoroquinolones [2,5].

5. MRSA and drug-resistant pathogen risk groups

Nemonoxacin's non-fluorinated C-8-methoxy quinolone structure underpins potent activity against Gram-positive pathogens, including **MRSA**, **MSSA**, and **penicillin-resistant Streptococcus pneumoniae**. Clinical experience in **skin and soft tissue infections (SSTI)**, supported by microbiology studies and post-marketing surveillance in China and Taiwan, shows:

- High microbiological activity against MRSA and other resistant Gram-positive organisms [2]
- Clinical cure rates in SSTI cohorts are comparable to established agents such as linezolid (where comparator data are available)
- No clear resistance-emergence signal over the surveillance period [2]

The document distills this into a concise takeaway:

"Nemonoxacin retains potent activity against MRSA and other resistant Gram-positive pathogens, with clinical outcomes consistent across high-risk groups."

These data reinforce Nemonoxacin's role in settings where resistant Gram-positive pathogens are prevalent [2] [4].

6. High pneumonia severity (PSI III–IV)

Moderate-to-severe community-acquired pneumonia (CAP) is where many antibiotics struggle to maintain consistent performance. In Nemonoxacin's Phase III CAP trials and Phase IV real-world studies, subgroup analyses of patients with **Pneumonia Severity Index (PSI) class III–IV** showed:

- Preserved clinical efficacy compared with the overall trial population

- A lower incidence of QT prolongation relative to fluoroquinolone comparators [2,5]

The document captures this succinctly:

"Nemonoxacin maintains efficacy in moderate-to-severe CAP (PSI III–IV), supporting its use in higher-risk respiratory cohorts."

This subgroup anchors Nemonoxacin's positioning in higher-acuity respiratory infections [2].

7. Cardiovascular comorbidities

Given the cardiotoxicity concerns associated with fluoroquinolones, cardiovascular comorbidity is a clinically important lens. Pooled safety analyses and post-marketing pharmacovigilance did not reveal a clinically meaningful **QT-prolongation signal** with Nemonoxacin, even in patients with pre-existing cardiovascular disease.

As the document notes:

"Cardiovascular comorbidity does not appear to increase Nemonoxacin-associated QT risk."

This supports the use of Nemonoxacin in multimorbid patients where cardiac safety is a key consideration [2,5].

8. Prior fluoroquinolone exposure

In an era of rising antimicrobial resistance, cross-resistance between new agents and legacy fluoroquinolones is a major concern. Microbiological surveillance and CAP clinical datasets indicate:

- No consistent cross-resistance pattern between Nemonoxacin and fluoroquinolones
- Clinical outcomes that are not adversely affected by prior fluoroquinolone exposure

These observations support Nemonoxacin's use in settings with high historical fluoroquinolone utilization [2].

9. Transplant patients: Small numbers, high relevance

Although the numbers are small, **case reports** and post-marketing pharmacovigilance in liver and kidney transplant recipients provide an important signal:

"No major safety concerns reported. No drug–drug interactions with calcineurin inhibitors identified."

Even low-N data can be meaningful in immunocompromised populations, particularly when they align with the broader PK and safety profile observed in other high-risk groups [2].

What these subgroups reveal about the molecule

Across all special populations, a consistent pattern emerges:

- **Stable PK** in most groups, with a clear, model-based adjustment strategy only in severe renal impairment [1]
- **Predictable safety**, including in the elderly, mild–moderate hepatic impairment, and patients with cardiovascular comorbidities [2]
- **Absence of hallmark fluoroquinolone liabilities**, such as dysglycemia and prominent QT-prolongation signals [2]
- **Sustained efficacy** across comorbidities, high-severity CAP, and resistant Gram-positive pathogen risk groups [2,4]

This chapter shows that Nemonoxacin's real-world performance is not defined by isolated anecdotes but by a **coherent, cross-population stability** that reinforces its clinical identity.

Chapter 13 told the story of the **first real-world signals** - the molecule's initial encounter with clinical reality. Chapter 14 now expands that story into **mature real-world performance**, showing how the molecule behaves across the full diversity of patients it ultimately serves.

Together, these chapters complete the transition from **controlled trials → early signals → broad clinical use**, forming the backbone of the molecule's real-world narrative.

Reference list for Chapter 14

1. **Li Y, Lu J, Kang Y, et al.** Nemonoxacin dosage adjustment in patients with severe renal impairment based on population pharmacokinetic and pharmacodynamic analysis. *Br J Clin Pharmacol.* 2021;87(10):4030-4043. doi:10.1111/bcp.14881.

2. **Yuan J, Zhang X, Chen J, et al.** Safety of oral Nemonoxacin: A systematic review of clinical trials and postmarketing surveillance. *Front Pharmacol.* 2022;13:1067686. doi:10.3389/fphar. 2022.1067686.

3. **U.S. Food and Drug Administration.** Guidance for Industry: Pharmacokinetics in Patients with Impaired Renal Function - Study Design, Data Analysis, and Impact on Dosing and Labeling. (Referenced for the regulatory framework underlying renal-impairment PK studies and dose-adjustment rationale.)

4. **Chen et al., Lauderdale et al., Demei et al.** Preclinical and microbiological studies describing the antibacterial spectrum of Nemonoxacin against Gram-positive cocci, including penicillin-resistant *S. pneumoniae* and MRSA, as cited in the systematic safety review and supporting its activity in MRSA/high-risk pathogen groups.

5. **Phase II/III, Phase IV, observational, and post-marketing datasets** summarized in Yuan et al. (2022), which provide the subgroup data for elderly, mild–moderate renal impairment, mild–moderate hepatic impairment, diabetes, cardiovascular comorbidities, PSI III–IV CAP, prior fluoroquinolone exposure, and transplant patients.

Chapter 15.

Territory Strategy and the Agreements Waiting for Their Time

The global expansion of Nemonoxacin has always been shaped not only by the territories where approvals were secured, but also by the regions where formal licensing agreements were established - agreements that opened doors, defined strategic intent, and positioned the molecule for future activation. These territories form a quiet but essential layer of the molecule's lifecycle architecture: options preserved, pathways mapped, and opportunities held in reserve.

Yet the journey also revealed a deeper truth: **even when agreements are signed, markets may not be ready**. Treatment guidelines, partner capability, regulatory maturity, and antimicrobial stewardship policies all influence whether a molecule can advance. The challenge is not merely scientific - it is one of positioning, timing, and alignment.

This chapter integrates those realities - and the strategies that may one day overcome them.

1. Latin America: A Region-Wide Agreement with Productos Científicos (2016)

In 2016, TaiGen entered a broad licensing agreement with Productos Científicos S.A. de C.V. (PC), covering Mexico, major South American markets, and Central American territories. The agreement granted PC exclusive rights to develop, register, and commercialize Nemonoxacin across the region.

Although no regulatory submissions have been initiated, the agreement remains intact. As Latin American healthcare systems modernize and antimicrobial resistance (AMR) burdens rise, the region may become increasingly receptive.

Strategic Pathways for Future Activation

- Target high-risk populations where narrow-spectrum antibiotics are insufficient.
- Use real-world evidence (RWE) from China to demonstrate safety and differentiation from traditional fluoroquinolones.
- Align with national AMR policies, positioning Nemonoxacin as a resistance-management tool rather than a first-line CAP drug.
- Phase-in market entry, beginning with hospital-based severe CAP risk groups.

These strategies transform the agreement from a dormant contract into a future-ready option.

2. Canada, Australia, and New Zealand: Commonwealth Markets under Luminarie Canada (2020)

The 2020 exclusivity agreement with Luminarie Canada Inc. covers three high-value Commonwealth markets. While no filings have been submitted, the agreement preserves access to jurisdictions with strong stewardship frameworks and high regulatory credibility.

Strategic Pathways for Future Activation

- Leverage RWE to address safety concerns associated with older fluoroquinolones.
- Position Nemonoxacin within AMR initiatives, especially as these countries strengthen stewardship policies.
- Explore niche indications (e.g., MRSA-risk CAP, quinolone-intolerant patients).
- Use Malaysia's NDA progress as a regional proof-of-concept.

These markets may move slowly, but once aligned, they can significantly amplify global credibility.

3. Southeast Asia: Agreements with Y.S.P. Industries (2023)

The 2023 agreement with Y.S.P. Industries (M) Sdn. Bhd. marked TaiGen's formal entry into Southeast Asia. In 2024, YSP submitted the NDA for Taigexyn® capsules to Malaysia's NPRA—an important milestone for the region.

Across many global markets, treatment guidelines for mild community-acquired pneumonia continue to favor narrow-spectrum antibiotics, reflecting stewardship priorities and cost-effectiveness considerations. This creates a common structural challenge for broad-spectrum agents: the risk of being perceived as “too strong” for mild disease, even when clinical need exists in specific subpopulations. This is not a country-specific dilemma but a recurring pattern in markets with mature stewardship frameworks.

Strategic Pathways Already in Motion

- Use the NDA review process as a demonstration of regulatory viability within Southeast Asia.
- Engage guideline committees with RWE and special-population data.
- Highlight the non-fluoroquinolone structure to differentiate from class-effect concerns.
- Position Nemonoxacin for high-risk CAP, where narrow-spectrum agents are insufficient.

Southeast Asia may become the region where the guideline barrier is first re-evaluated through evidence-based dialogue.

4. Vietnam: A Dual-Partner Model for Future Expansion (2025)

The 2025 agreement with Fideschem Inc. and Newsun Pharmaceutical JSC. grants 20-year rights in Vietnam. With one of the world’s highest AMR burdens and 270,000 AMR-related deaths between 2020 and 2023, Vietnam represents a market where clinical need is undeniable.

Strategic Pathways for Future Activation

- Frame Nemonoxacin as an AMR solution, not merely a CAP drug.
- Leverage Vietnam’s urgent public-health needs to accelerate regulatory engagement.

- Use the dual-partner structure to combine regulatory strength and distribution reach.
- Introduce hospital-first adoption, then expand to outpatient settings.

Vietnam may become a Southeast Asian anchor market alongside Malaysia.

5. The United States: A Retained Frontier

TaiGen retains full rights in the U.S. Although development has not advanced, evolving federal AMR incentives may reopen the pathway.

Strategic Pathways for Future Activation

- Monitor U.S. pull incentives (subscription models, PASTEUR Act).
- Position Nemonoxacin as a non-fluoroquinolone alternative, addressing class-effect concerns.
- Use global RWE to support future re-entry.
- Explore targeted indications requiring MRSA or resistant-pathogen coverage.

The U.S. remains the most significant - but also the most timing-dependent - option.

6. Agreements as Long-Duration Strategic Assets

Across all regions, the agreements share a common character: they are options, not outcomes. Their value lies in:

- Geographic optionality
- Regulatory optionality
- Partner optionality
- Lifecycle optionality

These agreements are structural beams in Nemonoxacin's long-term architecture - quiet, patient, and ready.

Transition to Chapter 16. Life-Cycle Management

These agreements reveal a deeper truth about global commercialization: a molecule's value is not defined solely by where it has launched, but by the foresight embedded in the territories it has prepared for. In the long arc of antibiotic lifecycle strategy, preserving optionality is as important as achieving early approvals. It is this interplay - between action and preparation, between realized markets and future horizons - that shapes the enduring relevance of an anti-infective.

Chapter 16 turns inward to examine the architecture that sustains that relevance: the intellectual, clinical, regulatory, and commercial structures that allow a molecule not only to enter the world, but to remain potent, protected, and strategically alive across decades.

PART V

Life-Cycle Strategy

This part ties everything together and shows how long-term value is engineered.

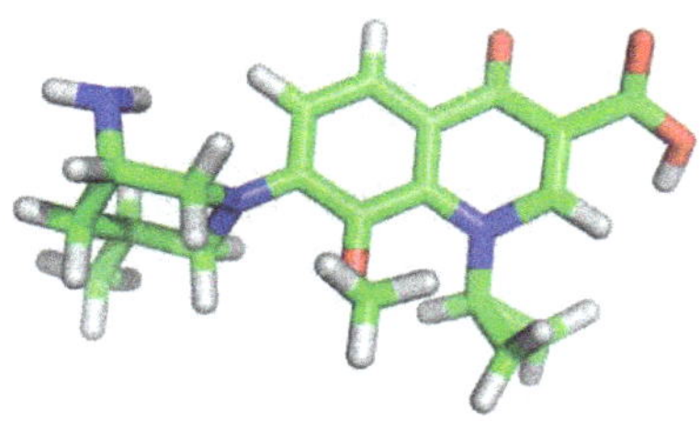

Chapter 16.

Life-Cycle Management

The life of an antibiotic does not begin with approval, nor does it end with the first commercial launch. For molecules like Nemonoxacin - born from decades of medicinal chemistry, refined through global clinical development, and carried across uneven regulatory landscapes - the true measure of endurance lies in what happens after the initial wave of scientific achievement.

Life-cycle management is the discipline that transforms a single approval into a multi-decade strategic asset. It is the craft that keeps the molecule ready for the opportunities described in Chapter 15 - especially in markets where guidelines, partner capability, or regulatory maturity have delayed progress.

1. The Philosophy of Enduring Value

TaiGen's life-cycle philosophy rests on three principles:

- Value must be layered.
- Adaptation must be continuous.
- Longevity must be intentional.

These principles are what allow Nemonoxacin to remain viable even in markets where positioning challenges - such as the "therapeutic overkill" dilemma - have slowed adoption.

2. Building Intellectual Architecture

A robust IP estate extending to 2042 enables:

- Re-entry into previously unready markets
- New indications for special populations
- Differentiation from traditional fluoroquinolones
- Protection of future formulations and delivery systems

This architecture is the backbone supporting all future BD strategies.

3. Clinical Evolution to Overcome Positioning Barriers

Many countries restrict first-line CAP treatment to narrow-spectrum antibiotics.

Life-cycle management provides the tools to overcome this with Clinical Strategies:

- Special-population studies (elderly, renal impairment, immunocompromised).
- MRSA-risk subgroup analyses to justify broader-spectrum use.
- Real-world evidence (RWE) demonstrating safety and low resistance induction.
- Post-marketing surveillance supporting guideline reconsideration.

These data directly address the concerns that have slowed BD progress.

4. Regulatory Renewal and AMR Alignment

Regulatory adaptation is essential for repositioning Nemonoxacin:

- Label updates incorporating new safety and population data.
- Alignment with AMR policies, reframing Nemonoxacin as a resistance-management tool.
- Preparation for pull incentives in the U.S. and Europe.
- Harmonization efforts enabling future filings in Latin America (LATAM), Commonwealth markets, and Southeast Asia.

Regulatory evolution becomes a strategic lever for overcoming guideline barriers.

5. Commercial Reinvention Across Markets

Commercial strategy is where life-cycle management meets real-world constraints.

Commercial Strategies:

- Hospital-first entry, avoiding guideline restrictions in outpatient mild CAP.
- Stewardship-aligned messaging, emphasizing safety and resistance profile.
- Partner diversification, ensuring no single market determines global fate.
- Re-evaluation of stalled markets, using Malaysia and Vietnam as demonstration cases.

These strategies allow Nemonoxacin to grow even when first-line CAP positioning is constrained.

6. Strategic Patience and the Long Game

TaiGen's approach recognizes that:

- Guidelines evolve slowly
- AMR crises accelerate policy change
- Partners mature over time
- Markets open in cycles

Life-cycle management is the discipline that keeps the molecule ready for these shifts.

7. Closing: A Molecule Prepared for the Future

With protection extending to 2042 and a deepening clinical and regulatory foundation, Nemonoxacin remains positioned for future relevance. Markets that were once inaccessible may open as AMR incentives strengthen. New partners may emerge with the capability to execute where others could not. And the global need for novel antibiotics will only intensify.

Life-cycle management ensured that Nemonoxacin did not fade after its first approvals. It preserved the molecule's potential, extended its value, and prepared it for opportunities that may arise years or even decades after its discovery. The art lies not in predicting the future, but in preparing a molecule to meet it.

PART VI

Reflections

The part that no regulatory filing or patent document can capture.

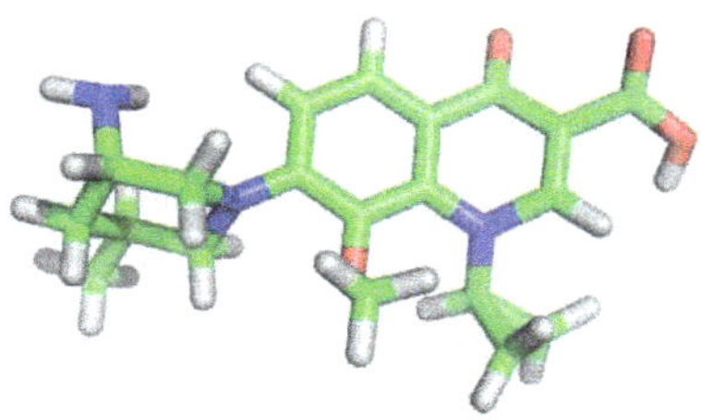

Chapter 17.

What the First Book Couldn't Tell

There are stories that can be told only once the dust has settled. When I wrote The Journey of Nemonoxacin, I believed I had captured the essential truth of the molecule's early life - the experiments, the failures, the improbable recoveries, and the people who carried it forward when the path was anything but clear. That book was my attempt to preserve the scientific memory before it faded: the bench work, the clinical puzzles, the sense of discovery that defined those years.

But even as I finished it, I knew there were parts of the story that did not fit within the frame of a scientific memoir. Some events were still unfolding. Some decisions were too entangled in ongoing negotiations. Some lessons were not yet lessons - only unresolved questions. And some truths could not be told until I had enough distance to understand them myself.

The first book could not tell how fragile a molecule becomes once it leaves the laboratory. It could not show the invisible forces that shape its fate: the patent claims that must be rebuilt, the regulatory pathways that diverge without warning, the commercial incentives that shift beneath your feet. It could not describe the moments when science was no longer the central challenge - when the real work was navigating systems that did not care about the molecule's promise, only about its compliance, its protection, its market logic.

Nor could it explain the emotional weight of those moments - the responsibility of carrying a molecule through institutions that were never designed to accommodate uncertainty, or the quiet fear that one misstep could erase years of work.

Most of all, I could not tell how my own understanding changed. In the early years, I believed that good science would speak for itself. That data, if honest and rigorous, would be enough. But the journey that followed taught me otherwise. I learned that innovation survives only when it is defended, translated, negotiated, and sometimes rescued. I learned that systems have their own tempos and their own blind spots. And I learned that guiding a molecule into the world requires a different kind of courage - one that is less visible, but no less demanding.

What the first book could not tell is what Chapters 15 and 16 finally make visible: that the world does not always move in synchrony with science.

Chapter 15 revealed the uneven readiness of global markets - the licensing agreements that opened doors but did not yet lead anywhere, the partners who hesitated because guidelines favored narrow-spectrum therapy, the perception that using a broad-spectrum agent for mild pneumonia was "therapeutic overkill." It showed how a molecule can be scientifically sound yet commercially stalled, not because it failed, but because the world around it was not ready. And it showed that even in stillness, these agreements were not failures but options - strategic footholds preserved for a future moment when clinical need, regulatory maturity, and partner capability finally align.

Chapter 16 turned inward to show how a molecule survives such uncertainty. It traced the architecture that keeps a drug alive across decades: the layered patents, the evolving clinical evidence, the regulatory adaptations, the stewardship-aligned positioning, and the strategic patience required to wait for markets to mature. It showed that life-cycle management is not a technical exercise but a philosophy - a way of ensuring that a discovery remains relevant long after its first approval, ready to re-enter markets that once seemed closed.

Together, these chapters tell the part of the story the first book could not: that the survival of a molecule is not guaranteed by science alone. It depends on strategy, timing, resilience, and the willingness to keep a door open even when no one is ready to walk through it.

This second volume exists because the scientific story was only half of the story. The other half lived in the spaces the first book could not reach: the strategy, the protection, the institutional battles, the decisions made under pressure, and the long, unglamorous work of ensuring that a discovery does not disappear before it has the chance to matter.

Together, the two books form a single arc. One captures the birth of an idea. The other captures its survival. And in the space between them lies the evolution of my own perspective - from scientist to steward, from observer to participant in the systems that determine whether a molecule becomes a medicine.

Chapter 18.

The Long Horizon

There comes a moment in every long project when the story stops being about the molecule alone and becomes a story about time. Not the urgent time of experiments or deadlines, but the slower, deeper time in which institutions evolve, markets shift, and scientific ideas either fade or find their place.

After the first book captured the birth of Nemonoxacin, and this volume traced its survival across systems that were never designed to move in harmony, the final question is no longer what happened, but what endures.

The long horizon is where a molecule's fate is no longer determined by the brilliance of its chemistry or the rigor of its trials, but by the patience to navigate uncertainty, the discipline to preserve optionality, and the willingness to continue shaping its relevance even when progress is invisible. It is the space where global agreements wait for their moment, where life-cycle strategies accumulate quietly, and where the work becomes less about breakthroughs and more about stewardship.

In this horizon, the story of Nemonoxacin is still unfolding. The markets that hesitated may yet open. The partners who paused may return with new capabilities. The policies that once constrained its positioning may shift under the weight of antimicrobial resistance. And the molecule itself - protected, studied, and continually reinterpreted - remains prepared for futures that could not have been imagined when the first experiments were run.

The long horizon also reveals something about the people who carry a molecule across decades. In the early years, the work is driven by discovery: the thrill of a new scaffold, the elegance of a synthetic route, the first glimpse of clinical promise. But as time passes, the work becomes quieter and more deliberate. It becomes the work of maintaining readiness, of defending value, of ensuring that a molecule does not disappear simply because the world has not yet caught up to it.

This is the part of the journey that rarely appears in scientific papers or regulatory dossiers. It is the part defined by conversations that lead nowhere until, suddenly, they do; by agreements that remain dormant until the world changes; by strategies that seem invisible until they become indispensable. It is the part where progress is measured not in milestones but in persistence.

And yet, this phase is not without its own form of discovery. It reveals the contours of global health systems, the inertia of guidelines, the fragility of commercial incentives, and the quiet power of evidence accumulated over time. It teaches that innovation is not a moment but a continuum - one that stretches far beyond the laboratory and into the shifting landscapes of policy, economics, and public health.

As Nemonoxacin enters this long horizon, its future is neither fixed nor finite. The molecule stands on a foundation strengthened by decades of work: a global IP estate extending to 2042, a clinical record that continues to deepen, regulatory pathways that remain open, and partnerships that hold the potential for renewal. Its journey is no longer defined by urgency, but by endurance.

Epilogue

The Legacy of a Molecule

When I look back across the two books that now frame the story of Nemonoxacin, I see more than a scientific achievement or a strategic accomplishment. I see a life's work - shaped by mentors, colleagues, skeptics, allies, and the quiet determination that carried us through uncertainty.

The first book captured the molecule's birth: the spark of discovery, the long nights in the lab, the clinical trials that tested its promise. It was the story of curiosity, persistence, and the belief that a new idea could matter.

This second book captures the molecule's survival: the patents that protected it, the regulatory systems that judged it, the commercial landscapes that challenged it, and the strategic decisions that allowed it to reach patients across continents. It is the story of translation - from science into law, from data into strategy, from innovation into impact.

Together, these books tell a single truth:

A molecule becomes a medicine only when science and strategy learn to speak to each other.

Nemonoxacin taught me that innovation is not a moment. It is a continuum - a sequence of choices, risks, revisions, and reflections. It taught me that systems matter as much as ideas, and that the people who navigate those systems shape the outcome as profoundly as the molecule itself.

Most of all, it taught me something about myself: that my work lives at the intersection of disciplines, cultures, and perspectives. That my role was not only to discover, but to define; not only to understand the science, but to protect it; not only to develop a molecule, but to guide it into the world.

But the lessons it offered will continue to shape the way I think, work, and lead.

And perhaps, someday, they will guide someone else - someone standing at the beginning of their own long, uncertain, extraordinary journey.

Acknowledgements

This second volume stands on a wider landscape than the first. While Book 1 captured the scientific origins of Nemonoxacin, this book traces its long arc across borders, institutions, regulatory systems, and decades of collective effort. It is therefore only fitting that my gratitude extends not only to the individuals who shaped the manuscript but also to the many teams whose work made the Nemonoxacin journey possible.

To those who made this book possible

I am deeply grateful to the colleagues who supported the reconstruction of timelines, regulatory histories, patent transitions, and clinical narratives that form the backbone of this volume. Their willingness to revisit documents, clarify details, and share institutional memory made it possible to tell this story with accuracy and integrity.

I also thank the many colleagues - past and present - who contributed materials, insights, and clarifications across the manuscript's development, especially in areas spanning China SFDA/NMPA submissions, Taiwan TFDA interactions, Russian MoH processes, and the evolution of the global patent portfolio.

To the scientific and functional teams behind Nemonoxacin

This book would not exist without the extraordinary teams whose work transformed Nemonoxacin from a promising molecule into a globally approved medicine. Book 2 documents their contributions in depth, and I wish to acknowledge them here with gratitude.

My thanks extend to the regulatory teams - Marie Chang, Dr. Yi-Jong Lin, Uwe Wu, Annie Bai, Tracy Wang, and others - whose diligence and persistence guided Nemonoxacin through complex, multi-jurisdictional pathways.

To the clinical development teams across Taiwan, China, and Russia - Dr. David Chung, Dr. Kit-Mui Chiu, Hao-Chen Tan, Dr. Hao

Zhang, Dr. Luke Lin, Dr. Chen-En Tsai, Zora Hsu, Alice Chen, Betty Li, Jenny Chang, Nina Chuang, Li-wen Chang, Dr. Guang-Yu Zhang, Dr. Pingping Jin, Xue-Wei Qiu, and many others—thank you for your unwavering commitment to scientific rigor and patient safety.

To the CMC, process chemistry, analytical chemistry, and technical operations teams - Dr. Shen-Yen Chou, Dr. Wen-Chang Chen, Judy Yuan, Dr. Jen Chrng, Te-Hsun Yang, Eric Wang, Kuo-Shu Peng - your work ensured that Nemonoxacin could be manufactured reliably, safely, and at scale across multiple countries and regulatory systems.

To the pharmacology, toxicology, and DMPK teams - Dr. Hua-Chien Chen, Dr. Shu-Jen Chen, Dr. Julius Huang, Dr. Paul Chow, Patty Huang, Dr. Gene Hsu, Dr. Ada Kung, Yumai Chen, Dr. Sophie Lee, Dr. Cheng-yuan Tsai - your foundational work established the scientific credibility that carried Nemonoxacin through global development.

To the Beijing operations team, led by Kuo-Lung Philip Huang, whose leadership in China's regulatory submission, SFDA dialogue, and clinical execution was essential to Nemonoxacin's success. Book 1 already recognized his contributions, and Book 2 further documents the depth of his impact.

To the patent and intellectual property teams, I extend special gratitude to Hossein Hakimelahi, whose expertise shaped the early patent strategy and protected the core composition claims, and to Xiao-Shan Xie of TaiGen Beijing, whose work supported the China-side patent and regulatory interface. Their contributions ensured that Nemonoxacin's scientific innovation was matched by a robust and enduring global patent estate.

To the Corporate Operations and Business Development teams - Joseph Hsush; Dr. Stephen Ip, Dr. John Jin, Dr. Gloria Hsieh, and Dr. Peter W. Tsao - thank you for the strategic coordination, partnership development, and organizational stewardship that shaped the molecule's path across the United States, Taiwan, China, Russia, and beyond. Your cross-border collaboration and strategic decisions were instrumental to the trajectory documented in this volume.

To the institutions and eras that shaped this journey

Nemonoxacin's story spans multiple organizations, acquisitions, and regulatory eras. I acknowledge with gratitude:

- TaiGen Biotechnology, and especially Dr. Min-Chu Hsu, the founder and CEO of TaiGen, whose vision and persistence carried Nemonoxacin from licensing to global commercialization.
- Procter & Gamble Pharmaceuticals, whose early discovery work and technology transfer laid the foundation for everything that followed.
- Zhejiang Medicine Co. Ltd. (ZMC), whose partnership enabled large-scale manufacturing and China NDA approvals.
- R-Pharm JSC, whose efforts brought Nemonoxacin to Russia and the CIS region.
- Regulatory agencies across Taiwan, China, Russia, and the United States, whose rigorous reviews shaped the drug's development and ensured its safety and efficacy.

These institutions collectively form the historical architecture of Nemonoxacin's journey.

Personal gratitude

My deepest thanks go to my family. To my wife, Lin-Shan King, whose steadfast support has accompanied every chapter of my professional life, and to my sons, Dr. Wilson King and Dr. Martin King, who once again offered thoughtful comments and encouragement during the preparation of this volume, as they did for Book 1.

Their presence has been a constant source of strength throughout the long arc of this two-volume work.

About The Author

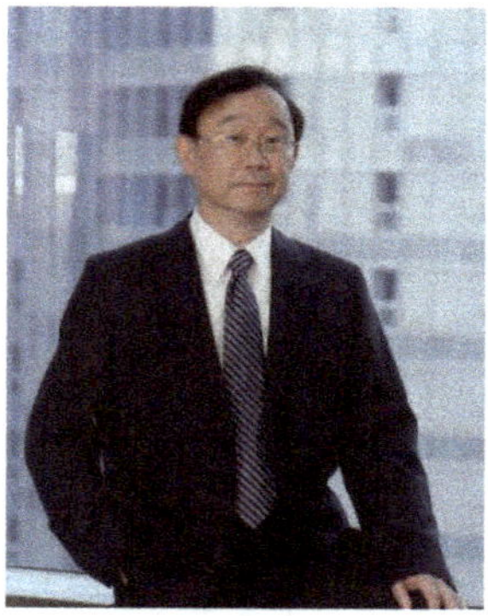

Chi-Hsin Richard King, Ph.D.

Dr. Chi-Hsin Richard King's career spans more than forty years and three continents, tracing a path from organic chemistry laboratories in Utah to boardrooms, clinical sites, and regulatory agencies across the United States, Taiwan, and China. Over these decades, he has helped shepherd new medicines from the earliest spark of an idea to global commercialization.

His work has touched every stage of drug development. He has guided molecules from in vitro discovery through IND submissions and multinational Phase I–III clinical trials. Along the way, he has authored 28 scientific papers, delivered 30 conference presentations, and built a portfolio of 34 patents covering treatments for pneumonia, antibiotic-resistant infections, stem-cell mobilization, major depressive disorder, hepatitis C, and influenza. Among these innovations is TG-1000, now approved in China as Pixavir marboxil - a milestone reflecting years of scientific and strategic effort.

Dr. King's leadership roles have positioned him at the forefront of influential biotechnology organizations. As Chief Scientific Officer at American BriVision Corporation (2017–2023) and Senior Vice President at TaiGen Biotechnology (2005–2017), he directed discovery research, CMC strategy, and global intellectual property initiatives. His oversight encompassed the development and commercialization of Nemonoxacin (Taigexyn®) as well as the discovery-stage advancement of TG-1000, shaping programs that bridged scientific innovation with worldwide therapeutic impact.

His earlier career at Albany Molecular Research Inc., the Industrial Technology Research Institute, Hoechst Marion Roussel, and The Dow Chemical Company shaped the broad scientific and managerial perspective he brings to his work.

Dr. King earned his Ph.D. in organic chemistry from the University of Utah and his B.S. in chemistry from National Taiwan Normal University. These foundations supported a lifetime devoted to scientific innovation and the pursuit of better medicines.

www.ingramcontent.com/pod-product-compliance
Lightning Source LLC
Chambersburg PA
CBHW071351230926
51846CB00002B/513
9781971588223